HARD GRAFT
OUR FIGHT AGAINST KILLER BLOOD

Hope you enjoy.
Mike

HARD GRAFT: OUR FIGHT AGAINST KILLER BLOOD

Copyright © 2023 Mike Niles
All rights reserved.

No part of this publication may be reproduced, stored in a retrieval system, or transmitted in any form or by any means, electronic, mechanical, photocopying, recording, scanning, or otherwise, without the prior written permission of the author.

Limit of Liability/Disclaimer of Warranty: This publication is designed to provide accurate and authoritative information in regard to the subject matter covered. It is sold with the understanding that neither the author nor the publisher is engaged in rendering legal, investment, accounting or other professional services. While the publisher and author have used their best efforts in preparing this book, they make no representations or warranties with respect to the accuracy or completeness of the contents of this book and specifically disclaim any implied warranties of merchantability or fitness for a particular purpose. No warranty may be created or extended by sales representatives or written sales materials. The advice and strategies contained herein may not be suitable for your situation. You should consult with a professional when appropriate. Neither the publisher nor the author shall be liable for any loss of profit or any other commercial damages, including but not limited to special, incidental, consequential, personal, or other damages.

ISBN: 9798851466854

Cover design by: Thomas D'Souza
First edition, 2023

Table of Contents

NEVER MISS A BEAT ... 7

CHAPTER ONE 12TH APRIL 1973 ... 10

A MOMENTOUS ATOMIC ACCIDENT OCTOBER 1958 ... 16

GROWING UP 1945-1966 ... 35

'THY BONE IS MARROWLESS' 1972 ... 41

FINDING THE SOURCE OF ALL LIFE 1963 ... 51

ANDREW BOSTIC 1970-1972 ... 66

CARING FOR SICK CHILDREN 1972 ... 81

LEAVE YOUR DEPOSITS AT THE BANK 1972 ... 102

SUPRESS YOUR INSTINCTS 1960 ... 109

ON THE EVE OF TRANSPLANT 12TH APRIL, 1973 ... 121

A HEALTH SERVICE FOR ALL 1972/73 ... 127

BOOM, BLAST AND RUIN 1973 ... 142

NEW IDEAS ARE NOT TO BE TRUSTED ... 157

THE TRANSPLANT ... 167

PERFECTING THE ART 1976 ... 179

A WORLD-FIRST, PERHAPS APRIL-AUGUST 1973 ... 189

THE ANSWERS WERE CLOSE-BY ALL ALONG MAY 1979 ... 204

CAUGHT BY SURPRISE 1981 220

NO STONE UNTURNED 1974 236

HANDING OVER THE BATON 1976 241

BIG DATA TO SOLVE A BIG PROBLEM 1980S 249

ANOTHER LIFE OVER TOO SOON 1978 262

ATTEMPTS TO RIGHT SO MANY WRONGS MID-1980S 271

MIND THE GAP 1993 283

WHAT HAPPENED NEXT? 302

AFTERWORD 319

Author's note

This is a work of nonfiction. Quotes and accounts are mostly derived from direct interviews and conversations with contributors but also from newspaper articles, diaries, letters, official reports and other documentation viewed in personal or public archives.

This book follows two distinct narratives: one of **Elisabeth Bostic** and her family's battle against a hidden disease in the 1970s. The other narrative outlines crucial scientific developments over centuries that brought Elisabeth and her family to this very point. Understanding and marvelling at the science (and scientists), even without specialist knowledge, allows us to appreciate how monumental a moment in history this was. To quote a character you'll soon meet, *"If scientific beauty cannot be enjoyed by an outsider, you haven't done a good enough job of explaining it."*

If some of the scientific narrative is a little confusing it's because our blood is a complex system. The interspersed chapters about the Bostic family story demonstrates how the science made a real-life difference. A timeline of events can be found at the back.

Characters in this book are real people, past and present. Some names have been changed to protect identity. All descriptions are based on true events but, where first-hand accounts are limited, informed creative licence fills the gaps.

About the author

Mike is founder of an award-winning non-profit organisation and author of the new book, Hard Graft. Originally from Doncaster, in Yorkshire, he has spent over a decade working in the charity sector in the UK.

A trained journalist, Mike enjoys interviewing experts on weird and wonderful topics with a view to bringing complex stories to a wider audience. He enjoys reading historical nonfiction that brings to life inspiring people's experiences, something he found in spades in the history of bone marrow transplantation.

Hard Graft captures a moment in time; an important story that has never been told before.

HARD GRAFT: OUR FIGHT AGAINST KILLER BLOOD

Never miss a beat

In the last few minutes your heart has been quite busy. Perhaps you've been making a cup of tea, boarding a train or getting ready for bed. In that time, without you really noticing, it has blasted 20 quarts of blood out from the left ventricle, through the aortic valve, and onto a long and winding journey through a complicated web of arteries around your body ranging in thickness from the size of a forefinger to the width of a single hair[1]. We're talking about a significant volume of blood. To put in context, if you walked into your local pub and asked the person behind the bar to line up 33-pints of beer, they'd prepare roughly the same amount of fluid that your heart distributes in just 240-seconds – or four minutes. It means that your little heart, the size of a clenched fist located slightly left of centre in your chest, is a robust piece of kit. It rhythmically pumps out this lifegiving beat 100,000 times every single day equating to approximately two-billion beats in an average lifetime.

And it packs a punch.

Each heartbeat produces around 1.3 Watts of energy and sends oxygen-starved red blood cells on their way to the lungs. Once there, these blood cells grab a heap of essential oxygen molecules – 100-

---

[1] Just a minute: incredible numbers at play at the macro and micro level (nih.gov)

million of them each, to be precise - and this now oxygen-rich blood continues its journey to all corners of our being, sustaining our metabolism and keeping things ticking over nicely.

There are other cells in the blood fluid too that don't bother themselves with oxygen. Around 50-billion white blood cells join the rough and tumble journey through our body's 96,000 kilometres of arteries, veins and capillaries forming a highly technical surveillance of the entire system. They're swimming along in an ultra-rich liquid nutrient on high alert, surveilling the body looking for issues. Their job is to keep us healthy and, should they see an invader – such as a virus – be ready to step in if called upon.

Blood's journey doesn't begin in the heart, though. That's the powerful engine room. As the existing flow circulates it picks up new passengers along the way; fresh blood cells manufactured inside the body's own blood factories ready to get to work. These production lines are found in the middle of our bones, a fatty substance called the marrow, and they keep themselves extremely busy. Every single second - asleep or awake - these factories create two to three million new red blood cells. That rate of production may seem a little excessive but it's actually pretty important. Every minute sees the death of around 300-million of our cells.

Yet despite how intensely the engine room works, and no matter how relentlessly the factory delivers fresh stock, sometimes the blood is a little faulty.

This story focuses on what happens when there is a glitch in the system. When the micro processes that give us life, and protect us from harm, start to malfunction. It could impact any of us. It can tear families apart or bind them closer. Defeat medical minds or sharpen them. Reaffirm life or end it.

The chapters you're about to read shimmy between dogged efforts to advance treatment and the real-life consequences on people. A look into a melee of mesmerising wisdom and incredible individual courage along with heaped teaspoons of blind luck. We traverse our planet for crucial moments: from Staithes to Seattle, Belgrade to Bari, Middlesbrough to the Mekong Delta, Wisconsin to Westminster. The stories feature mothers and fathers, doctors and nurses, siblings and strangers, scientists and soldiers.

If you fit one of those roles, or even if you don't, this story is relevant. It could happen to any of us.

As humans, our reliance on healthy blood is absolute. Mysteries inside our circulatory system have baffled the greatest scientific and medical minds for centuries and, until very recently, the glitches signified unavoidable death.

In the 1960s, a child diagnosed with a severe immune deficiency had just a one in 10 chance of surviving childhood. With such limited understanding, the unknowns of our white blood cells meant an almost certain death sentence.

By the end of the 1980s, however, a child diagnosed with the very same blood disease could expect a nine in 10 chance of surviving and living to adulthood[i,ii].

So, what happened in those 30 years?

From a place of no hope, drastic change required a brand-new belief system. At a time of perilous danger, to abandon hope of a miracle and put faith in a stranger.

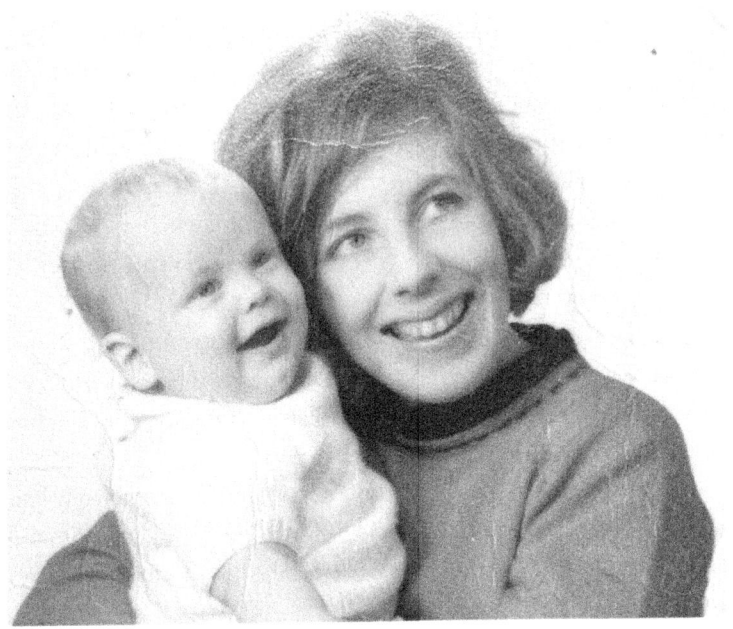

CHAPTER ONE
12th April 1973

Warm evening bustle spilled from the little pub on the corner. Conversation hummed from bunched groups as fixed lines blurred; strangers becoming friends and then strangers again. Wood panelled walls, saturated with the smells of years, boxed-in humid warmth. Mosaic windowpanes framing the scene condensed, inner breath colliding with cooled glass, chilled by the brisk London evening.

Roger hopscotched the worn, patterned carpet as he returned from the bar, snatching sips of his pint. The landlord pleased the thirsty crowd with dizzying speed; a familiar and unknowing comfort to

Roger as the months had progressed. By no means did Roger spent too much time in The Royal Oak. He didn't seek refuge at the bottom of a pint pot, drinking a tough day into the past, numbing the prospect of the next. But those times he had popped in, his demeanour struck the landlord as taut but calm. He'd always offered a kindly and unjudgmental welcome. Roger silently appreciated that. Dodging bar stools and flailing arms, Roger made his way to the corner table, thick-rimmed glasses steaming up with no available hands to wipe. His wife, Elisabeth, and her parents, keenly guided the drinks in, semaphore with their eyes.

It had been a draining day, something all too familiar. The foursome squeezed themselves into a congested corner, seeking quiet in a busy place. An emotional vice had progressively tightened around them for over two-years, squeezing out innocence. The younger couple looked tired for it.

Conversation felt forced. Liz, as she preferred to be known, jabbed the end of a cigarette into the glass ash tray. She was particularly restless. Her slight, wiry frame perched forward on the knee-high bar stool, agitated and uneasy. She was exhausted. Lazy ringlets of tired-looking hair drooped over her shoulders. That first gin and tonic had calmed the nerves.

Liz lit another cigarette. Her new pack of Woodbines was suddenly half empty. She wasn't alone, thick plumes coming from all corners, bouncing from beam to beam along the ceiling; the cloudy pub air congealed, as if something you could squeeze. She exhaled a fresh drag with eyes closed.

Denis, her father, fiddled nonsensically with Tetley's beer mats on the table, occasionally flipping and catching, trying always to land monocle side up. David Bowie was ballading on the pub speakers in the background, 'Drive-In Saturday'. Denis didn't have much time for all this modern music, he preferred classical. More Puccini and

Elgar than Pink Floyd and Elvis. He was a slender, moustachioed man who'd seen a lot in his time. A silent type: short in stature at just 5'4, this wasn't really his scene, more comfortable having a night in than drinking in a busy London pub.

Attempting a distraction from the strain of reality, his wife Mollie shared a story about the next-door-but-one neighbours in rural North Mymms taking their grandson on a trip to London Zoo for his birthday. Utterly insignificant, given the circumstances, but irrelevance was a welcome reprieve. She was exhausting all avenues of small talk. Normally shy and introverted, Mollie was desperate to distract her daughter's attention. She'd already covered their trip to the polling station that morning as the country elected representatives for new local authorities for the first time. They were there when the polls opened, casting their vote early to get into London as soon as possible.

Liz rocked on her cushioned stool. She knew what her mum was doing and was grateful. Uninterested and shattered, she let every boring detail wash over her. It filled a silent gap.

She was distracted. As things stood, the whole upcoming event was called off.

The whirr of the pub had grown, a new crowd making quite a fuss. Celebrating, perhaps. Liz had entirely forgotten today was voting day.

Still only half-listening, she directed a purposeful gaze to the bar. Cutting through the garbled hum was the smothered sound of a telephone. After handing coins to a customer, the landlord picked up the receiver. It had sounded for nine rings. Liz shot a glance around the table; no one else had noticed. No longer could she hear her mother's words, just saw her mouth rising and falling without sound; her attention had switched.

She knew this call was for her.

A few long seconds passed before, with a twist and gesture through the smoky haze, the landlord gave her the nod.

Pale lemons lay imperfectly sliced next to the ice bucket, each disagreed with the next in breadth and uniformity. How was it possible to slice a lemon so haphazardly? A shallow pool of rum lay idle on the wooden surface next to it, gathered drips from the optic above. She absorbed the mundane; her eyes fixating on dull distractions as she listened intently to the voice in her ear. Roger fixated on Liz.

Her body language transformed; rigid at first, the few words she spoke appeared stern. But her stance soon softened, shoulders melting south into her body. She clicked the receiver back onto its holster. A nod of appreciation in the direction of the landlord, too busy to notice. The clock had just passed nine-thirty.

"It's happening."

Abrupt and urgent, the table understood. She sunk the G&T in one, shook the rain from her coat and was waiting by the door before the others had even managed to stand. Ready for the weather they stepped into the square, a short journey through the cold and smokily damp night air in the shadows of the Houses of Parliament. Heel clicks fashioned a regular beat as, hands joined, Liz and Roger strode resolutely around the black iron railings, eagerly pursued by her parents. Light drizzle soaked the family, adding more weight to their day. What was about to happen? An overwhelming range of outcomes, yet she'd accept only one.

Liz recalled her exit a few hours before. It had been rather dramatic, loud and somewhat unbecoming, yet utterly essential. She envisioned the reception that might await her, awkward looks and uncomfortable conversations. She'd refuse to apologise. Curls now sodden, slick against her forehead, she squeezed Roger's hand; he continued looking straight ahead. Anticipation consumed them both.

A crowd of perhaps five journalists and photographers gathered at the base of the steps at the main entrance, insistent yet kind, as ever. News travels fast, it seemed. Liz knew the inevitability of this being a front-page scoop; not much new there. The papers wouldn't learn the full details until it was all over. Neither would she.

Liz exchanged a few nervous smiles; no time to chat. She began the ascent to the clammy warmth of the hospital and her family's destiny.

The chattering scrum muffled and then silenced behind closing doors. They took their well-trodden route along a marble-floored corridor before descending to the basement level. Liz led the way, flanked by the supporting cast; her stride purposeful, palms dry, face drawn. She'd caught a glimpse of her thin reflection in the pub toilets, each droop and crack depicting the strains, telling a story. Like candle wax aside a drained wine bottle; remnants hinting of glories past. No one knows the torment.

Approaching the office, she inspected her surroundings. Dark edges, the meeting place of wall and floor, served as a dust trap. Aged paint chipped and peeled from every surface. Not even *it* wished to be here. Yet she dreamed of being nowhere else. This shabby, run-down Victorian building, in a drab part of London, housed the single hope of keeping her son alive. Her *only* living son. After the death of her eldest, she now faced losing her youngest in identical circumstances.

Turning the corner, she met the gaze of the Professor, his eyes expectant and focused. Emotion rose from her core, shaking her almost to tears. "Everything we discussed is in place. Preparations are underway and the procedure will go ahead tomorrow. All we need now…"

Liz knew what he needed now. Her written consent. She gave it.

What was to take place had never been achieved before in medical history. It would be a ground-breaking world first; or not. It was the 'not' that she couldn't escape.

Her little boy blissfully slept, none-the-wiser, as she and Roger blew kisses through the glass and made their journey to their bedroom for the night. The parent flat was located on the top floor, still somewhat worn-out but a restful green oasis, enjoying fitted carpets and a few basic home comforts. Comparative luxury out-of-sync with the clinical coldness of her son's room below.

It was late when Mollie and Denis descended the hospital steps, heading home. A few reporters remained, chatting and smoking. There would be no news tonight, but they already knew that. A young journalist called Jane, who Mollie had become fond of over the weeks, drew alongside.

"I pray that it will be a lucky Friday the thirteenth for Simon tomorrow."

Mollie didn't believe in superstition but the comment paused her mid stride. She smiled at Jane for the briefest of seconds and continued to the car.

A momentous atomic accident
October 1958

There was nothing particularly extraordinary about this Wednesday morning aside from the fact that Života Vranić was going to be early into work. That's not to say he was *never* early but enthusiastic of newfound social circles, in the relative freedom his city now enjoyed, meant early mornings were not his forte. An advanced student of physics at the Faculty of Science, Belgrade University, Života had landed a coveted role working at the exciting new nuclear research institute on the banks of the River Danube. Honing a fledgling career at the jewel in the crown of the Yugoslav nuclear research programme was a pretty strong way to begin his journey. Života felt he had the city to himself as he cycled through a quiet Republic Square anticipating the day's schedule. Glancing at the clock up above the entrance of the bank it displayed 07:05.

The institute where Života worked, located in Vinča just south of the capital city of Belgrade, was the result of an unparalleled decade of investment in nuclear power for the young Yugoslav state. For many, Vinča itself was regarded as paramount to an ambitious program of nuclear research, led by President Josip Broz Tito, and nervous onlookers believed it consistent with developing capability to build an atomic bomb[iii]. The leader's very public fall-out with

Stalin, and growing acknowledgement of the Soviet nuclear weapon plans, may have spurred this momentous drive. Unsurprisingly the U.S., among others, were keeping a close eye on the progress of young Života and his colleagues.

We find ourselves in the decade-or-so-old Federal People's Republic of Yugoslavia. Citizens experienced wholesale change in the years after World War II, with the monarchy abolished and newly empowered President launching the sizeable task of rebuilding infrastructure and spirit of a city and nation. He envisioned a Yugoslavia that would prominently feature on the global stage and nothing, at this time, quite spoke of power like nuclear.

This radioactive scene, in the former Eastern Bloc, is in the autumnal months of 1958. We will soon see why Vinča would be an important moment in the history of blood disease but, for a little nuclear context, we need to take a leap back to the turn of the 20th century.

Splitting the atom

By now, scientists had realised that everything on earth was made up of tiny little things called atoms - derived from the Greek word 'atomos', which means indivisible. To demonstrate the relative size, if every atom in a human hand was the size of a marble the hand itself would be the size of Earth. Put another way, it is believed that there are more stars in the known Universe than grains of sand on all the beaches in the world. Yet a single grain of sand contains more atoms than the total number of stars[2].

---

[2] It's estimated there are around 43 quintillion atoms per grain of sand, in case you wanted to know.

They really are very small.

In 1897, British physicist Joseph John Thompson determined that within an atom was an even smaller particle which he called an 'electron', holding a negative electrical charge. Thompson explained that it orbited the central nucleus of the atom, like the earth around the sun. And that's all we knew about atoms until a few years later, in 1905, when a young scientist working in a factory in Bern, Switzerland, developed a theory that changed everything.

Albert Einstein, then just 26 years old, produced his now famous formula $e=mc^2$ determining that energy (e) was equal to mass (m) multiplied by the speed of light (c) squared. Einstein believed that physical matter, in whatever form, contained huge amounts energy stored up within its atoms. The problem was, he had no idea how to access it, or if that was even possible (remember, they thought it was impossible to divide atoms). But Einstein recognised a vast potential: solve this problem and you could unlock a significant source of 'free' and unending energy.

With such a tantalizing prospect, scientists set to work focusing on the nucleus where they believed this mysterious energy to be stored. Pretty soon, New Zealand scientist, Ernest Rutherford, found smaller parts within the nucleus, namely a proton (positive charge), a neutron (no charge, or neutral charge) and electrons (negative charge) orbiting around. The interesting particle here was the neutron. With no charge it didn't repel other particles when scientists fired much smaller sub-atomic particles at it. They did this to try and deconstruct the element; smash it up to see if they could transform the particle into something new and unique – and it worked. The experiments were yielding results and in 1934, the French chemist Irène Joliot-Curie (daughter of Marie Curie) and her husband, Frédéric Joliot-Curie, announced that they'd 'bombarded' elements with alpha particles and induced radioactivity in them.

Radioactivity, the term for the process by which an unstable atomic nucleus loses energy and decays by radiation, won them the Nobel Prize in Chemistry the following year. Despite their efforts, no 'unending energy source' just yet.

We've suddenly got very technical but bear with it.

Next up was Italian physicist, Enrico Fermi, who made it his daily task to fire particles at the atoms of different elements using radiation. A little niche, sure, but he was observing any transformations, trying to find this theoretical energy store. Starting with platinum, an element with a high atomic number, he had no success. He then bombarded aluminium neutrons, which successfully broke down into sodium and then decayed into magnesium. OK, he thought, now we have some progress. Fermi and his team of scientists worked their way through the periodic table, one-by-one and element-by-element, to see how the reactions differed. Now, it's unlikely these guys had people hanging on their every word at a party but they were painstakingly systematic and boisterously excited about splitting something 10,000x smaller than an atom (which, we've already discovered, is mind-bogglingly small). And, it turns out, they were onto something.

They methodically continued until they eventually reached the heaviest element, Uranium. Now things get interesting. There was a reaction but, unusually, they were unable to determine or explain the end product, producing a never-before-seen element with radioactive properties. Nevertheless, they published their results and Fermi was awarded the Nobel Prize for demonstrating 'the existence of new radioactive elements produced by neutron irradiation'.

Enrico Fermi was to receive his coveted 1938 prize in Stockholm on 10th December and made a request to the Italian Government, which was approved, for special dispensation allowing his whole family to travel with him to receive this great honour. But the group trip was about more than family pride. Earlier that year, newly introduced racial laws were promulgated by Italian President, Benito Mussolini, to bring Italian Fascism ideologically closer to German National Socialism. This threatened the freedoms of Fermi's Jewish wife, Laura, so after the ceremony the couple, along with their two children, left King Gustavus V and the Concert Hall behind and promptly disappeared into the dark Stockholm night to set off on their secretly planned escape for New York. He was joining many prominent European scientists that had already made the decision to flee for the United States including Einstein, himself of German Jewish descent.

Over on the other side of Sweden, in the western town of Kungälv, as Fermi made final preparations to vanish across the Atlantic Ocean, the physicist Lise Meitner sat at her dressing table reading a letter she'd just received from a scientific peer in Germany. Until earlier that year, Vienna-born Meitner had worked as head of the physics department of the Kaiser Wilhelm Institute (KWI) for Chemistry in Berlin but, following the annexation of her native Austria into Nazi Germany in March, was no longer safe. In a prominent and visible position, she'd found herself in immediate danger and fled.

The letter she read was written by a former colleague, Otto Hahn; a chemist she'd worked closely alongside and collaborated with for many years at the institute. They considered themselves friends, the Hahn and Meitner Laboratories had been the leading branches at the KWI for Chemistry and they'd been jointly nominated multiple times in the 1920s for the Nobel Prize for Chemistry. Prior to fleeing Germany, Hahn placed his mother's diamond ring in her possession in case it was needed for bribery crossing borders. After a perilous journey, she was welcomed as a scientific refugee in Sweden; one of the few remaining countries to accept her Austrian passport.

Meitner and Hahn safely reconnected a few months later, on 13th November, at a science summit in Copenhagen. Proudly showing Meitner his uranium research, she quickly dismissed his findings. It was clear to her that something wasn't quite correct and that his experiments must be re-done. He took her advice and now, in this correspondence, claimed the element barium resulted from bombarding uranium with neutrons.

Fresh questions fizzed through her mind. Could this be *it*? After reviewing the paperwork Meitner, along with her nephew and scientist Otto Frisch, visiting from Denmark, took a walk. As the story goes it was a blustery snowy December evening in Kungälv and the pair set off pondering Hahn's latest findings, Frisch on his skis and Meitner on-foot (claiming, correctly, she could travel just as fast).

They couldn't get their heads around the outcome. Barium has an atomic mass 40% less than uranium and radioactive decay could not possibly account for such a large difference in the mass of the nucleus. Resting on a tree trunk they jotted down rushed calculations on scraps of paper they found in their pockets. It was here they made the leap; if the split led to one part being barium, as Hahn had claimed, then their estimates meant the other part must be krypton. The combined mass of the two was slightly less than the original uranium atom so, according to Einstein's energy and mass formula, that gap must have resulted in an energy release. Meitner estimated a sizeable energy release[iv]; as it turns out, the most powerful energy source ever discovered.

Frisch termed this process 'nuclear fission', based on his knowledge of binary fission in biology; the asexual reproduction (or split) of cells in organisms like amoeba and bacteria. By understanding the fission process of a uranium nucleus, Meitner, Frisch and Hahn had unlocked a potentially unending natural energy source that would lead to great highs and great lows in human history[v].

A very close call

OK, that was a lot of detailed science to understand how nuclear energy came to be so, before we go on, let's have a little reprieve and consider, for a second, how vastly different our world could be now had a few moments in history played out slightly differently.

Imagine realising that the obscure element, uranium, has the potential to generate huge amounts of energy. While this could be used to power hundreds of thousands of households with electricity, the scientists also realised its potential, if harnessed, to destroy an entire city. Then imagine this discovery has been made in 1938 Germany under the watchful eye of Adolf Hitler.

In the months leading up to Hahn's experiment, passports of German Jews had been declared invalid (October), Kristallnacht had occurred killing 91 Jews and destroying synagogues (November) and in December, the same month as the discovery, the first Kindertransport arrived in Britain carrying unaccompanied children sent by desperate parents in the hope they would avoid persecution. The situation was escalating in Germany and, as word spread in science circles about the nuclear fission discovery, European scientists, many now based in the U.S., were all too aware of the danger it could pose in the wrong hands.

Not wishing to sound like a cliché line from a Hollywood movie, this group of experts decided they needed to warn the President. Without urgent action, an atomic bomb could be in the possession of the Nazis and, while World War II was still a few years away, signs of imperialist strategy were already becoming clear. European scientists in the U.S., including Enrico Fermi, set about raising the alarm but authorities were initially a little tone-deaf to the appeals of foreign experts speaking in thick accents and broken English. They needed a new approach, deciding this message of "extremely powerful bombs of a new type" needed to come from someone more recognisable. In September 1939, President Franklin D. Roosevelt opened a letter at his desk in the Oval Office from celebrity scientist, Albert Einstein. The letter had the desired impact and a new research programme was funded to get ahead of the game. The race had begun.

"No more Matilda's"

Interpretations scribbled on scrap pieces of paper in a Swedish snowstorm were beginning to have sizeable reactions on the other side of the world. Lise Meitner's calculations, based on the experiments conducted by her colleague, Otto Hahn, were to ignite a pursuit for nuclear power that continues to this day[vi].

So why, if Meitner identified the power of this process, was Hahn later awarded a Nobel Prize for Chemistry for the discovery of nuclear fission and not her (and Frisch)? Meitner herself wrote: 'Surely Hahn fully deserved the Nobel Prize for chemistry. There is really no doubt about it. But I believe that Otto Robert Frisch and I contributed something not insignificant to the clarification of the process of uranium fission - how it originates and that it produces so much energy and that was something very remote to Hahn.'

Despite obstacles denying women the same access to education as men, the field of science was somewhat of an equalizer, in some ways ahead of other professions in terms of gender equality. That is not to say that women were recognised comparably to men publicly with only two women awarded Nobel prizes in science or medicine between 1901-1963, both being Curie's[vii]. In the lab, however, many women of science were respected equals among male peers, primarily owing to the very matter of fact results that science demands. The road to this point, however, hadn't been a bed of roses.

In 1636, Dutch scholar Anna Maria van Schurman was the first woman ever allowed to attend university lectures but, curiously, was forced to sit behind a screen so that her fellow male students wouldn't see her. A few years later in nearby France, Martine Bertereau, the first female mineralogist, found herself imprisoned on suspicion of witchcraft after publishing two written works on the science of mining and metallurgy (researching the properties and purification of metals) before being arrested. That's right, witchcraft. A breakthrough came in 1732 as Italian physicist, Laura Bassi, at the age of 20 was enrolled as the first female member of the Bologna Academy of Sciences. One month later, she publicly defended her academic thesis and received a PhD. Bassi was awarded an honorary position as professor of physics at the University of Bologna becoming the first female physics professor in the world.

Now we're getting somewhere.

In the 1840s the British mathematician and scientist, Ada Lovelace, wrote a mathematical algorithm making her the world's first computer programmer. In 1874, Julia Lermontova was the first Russian woman to receive a doctorate in chemistry and in 1888, the American chemist, Josephine Silone Yates, was appointed head of the Department of Natural Sciences at the Lincoln Institute and, in so becoming, was the first Black woman to head a college science department in the United States.

Discoveries and achievements of women in science were increasingly widespread but many notable contributions, as in the case of Lise Meitner, were overlooked or not credited when it mattered. This was coined *The Matilda Effect*; a trend first described by suffragist Matilda Joslyn Gage as the bias against acknowledging the achievements of women scientists and, instead, attributing them to male colleagues[3].

Relevant to our story of blood disease, British chemist Rosalind Franklin's contribution to the discovery of DNA structures, in the 1950s, was one such instance. Franklin, and her graduate student Raymond Gosling, were trying to identify the configuration of heredity when they took a now infamous x-ray, Photo 51. It showed the composition better than anyone had done before with Franklin commenting 'the results suggest a helical structure'. Unbeknownst to Franklin, the image was shared with chemists from rival institution Cambridge University, Francis Crick and James Watson, who went on to develop the double helix theory of DNA structure. At no point did they credit Franklin or Gosling's contributions. She died a few years later, at the age of just 37, and the men went on to be awarded the Nobel Prize for one of the most important scientific discoveries of the 20th century. Another hidden hero of the DNA journey is Florence Bell. An X-ray crystallographer at the University of Leeds, she presented novel notions of DNA as an ordered structure back in 1938, way before Franklin, like a 'pile of pennies'. It contributed foundational thinking but, leaving scientific research after World War II, her contributions were almost entirely forgotten

---

[3] A famous case is geneticist Nettie Stevens who discovered sex chromosomes but her more renowned male colleague was credited with the discovery.

until recent efforts to give her appropriate credit[4].

The decision to ignore a woman's contribution, on account of her being a woman, is something that history has time and again shown to be a grave mistake. Except, that is, in the fortunate case of Ida Noddack.

In 1934, the chemist published a paper, 'On Element 93', in which she challenged Enrico Fermi's claims that he'd discovered an element with a higher atomic number than uranium. "It is conceivable', she wrote, 'that the nucleus breaks up into several large fragments, which would of course be isotopes of known elements but would not be neighbours of the irradiated element." That is to say that smashing up and splitting the uranium nucleus would result in other elements forming and perhaps with unusual results.

This paper was just a theory, without experimental proof, meaning it went largely ignored by leading scientists at the time, including Fermi. She even wrote to him personally suggesting he look at it again, to no avail. Noddack's theory never really saw the light of day. What Noddack had in fact proposed here, before anyone else, was nuclear fission.

Forget Einstein and the group of European scientists dramatically rushing to warn the President that the Nazis could blow up a city. It would have been way too late. If Noddack's theory had been listened

---

[4] A few scientists noticed the sexism in their field. Pathologist Frieda Robscheit-Robbins was, in the view of her colleagues, excluded from receiving a shared Nobel Prize in 1934 for her work on treating anaemia. Co-author of 21 papers on the topic of liver tissue as a treatment she would have become the second woman in history to receive the award after Marie Curie. When Robscheit-Robbins' male colleagues received the award, George Whipple shared his prize money and notoriety equally with her. Taking this a step further, microbiologist Elizabeth Lee Hazen, and her biochemist colleague Rachel Fuller Brown, filed a patent in 1950 for nystatin: an antifungal medication. Once awarded in 1957, the pair donated their royalties, over $13 million, to a trust fund for science and advancing women in science.

to, and worked on, at the time she published her paper, Germany could have gained a five-year head start on the rest of the world in the pursuit of nuclear weapons[5]. A slight change of events could have seen the bombs falling on London and Coventry and Glasgow filled with a nuclear material. The Blitz could have, in fact, seen the use of hundreds or thousands of atomic bombs. Devastation could have rained down on Britain before the Allies had a clue how to even split the atom.

As it turned out, the Lise Meitner and Otto Hahn's discovery made the development of the 'A-bomb' a realistic possibility. President Roosevelt's $600 million commitment was named 'The Manhattan Project' with the aim of manipulating the potential of nuclear fission for use in warfare before anyone else.

Over the next six years, Enrico Fermi and the European scientists worked on the chemistry while theoretical physicist, J. Robert Oppenheimer, was drafted in to design the bomb.

At 08:15 on the morning of 6th August 1945, bombardier Major Thomas Ferebee released the 'Little Boy' missile containing 64 kg (141 lb) of uranium-235 above the Japanese city of Hiroshima. Forty-four seconds later the atomic bomb detonated directly over a local hospital creating that infamous image of a huge mushroom cloud into the sky. Approximately 70–80,000 people, around 30% of the population of Hiroshima at the time, were killed by the blast and resultant firestorm, another 70,000 were injured.

In a radio address, President Harold Truman, now in position after the death of President Roosevelt, announced the U.S. use of the atomic bomb, claiming they'd targeted a military base. He stated "we

---

[5] The German government formed a secret committee in 1939 with a view to creating a nuclear weapon five years after Ida Noddack's theory was published.

won the race of discovery against the Germans" – albeit with a lot of German scientists contributing to his outcome.

Three days later, on 9th August 1945, pilot Charles W. Sweeney positioned his Bockscar aircraft over the Japanese city of Nagasaki where a second, stubby looking bomb, named 'Fat Man', was dropped. Up to 40,000 people instantly died and a few days later the Japanese government agreed to the terms of surrender, knowing that the U.S. had more atomic bombs ready to drop in September and October.

Otto Hahn heard the news of the Hiroshima atomic bomb from his location at Farm Hall where he was detained as a prisoner of war, along with nine other scientists, by the British forces. As the war ended, the scientists remained prisoners just outside Cambridge, codenamed Operation Epsilon, where intelligence agents aimed to learn how close the Germans were to constructing an atomic bomb of their own. "I thank God on my bended knees that we did not make a uranium bomb", Hahn was heard saying via hidden microphones, devastated and suicidal that his discovery had cost so many lives. "I wanted to suggest that all uranium should be sunk to the bottom of the ocean." Meitner had, in fact, been approached by the U.S. Government to work for them on developing nuclear weapons, but she flat-out refused, declaring: "I will have nothing to do with a bomb!"[6]

The power of nuclear fission had been categorically demonstrated to a global audience. The war over, attention turned to the energy it created and the self-sustaining chain reaction as a possible source of domestic power.

---

[6] Sime, Ruth Lewin (1996). Lise Meitner: A Life in Physics. Berkeley: University of California Press. ISBN 978-0-520-08906-8. OCLC 32893857

Energy from an atom

Back to the Autumnal morning of 15th October 1958 and Života Vranić approached the end of his cycle commute at the RB research reactor, one of two reactors at the Vinča site. Situated on the edge of town, completely separated from the thriving streets of the city, the power station cast an isolated figure against a grey backdrop of fields and sky.

The bright and acutely focused research team consisted of six personnel. Twenty-four-year-old Života was conducting an experiment for his graduation thesis where the reactor initiated a fission nuclear chain reaction. Everything gets incredibly hot; kinetic energy and gamma rays become thermal energy, to the tune of three million times higher than burning the same weight of coal fuel. As with most days at the plant the practical tasks were planned out ahead in every detail with tests taking place on the reactor. His exciting role pitted his skills alongside some great minds including Rosanda Dangubić, Radojko Maksić, Draško Grujić, Stijepo Hajduković and Živorad Bogojević.

As the time approached 10am consensus rippled through the group that ozone could be smelt in the air. It's not a good sign. Ozone, scientifically known as trioxygen due to it comprising of three oxygen atoms, is notably pungent in odour with a smell often described as similar to that of chlorine. Without warning the readings for the reactor suddenly became jammed. Scales that should demonstrate levels of radioactivity all displayed unreadable measures sending the young and inexperienced team into panic. There was a delay. The students were not trained to deal with such a situation and it took around ten minutes to identify the source.

The reactor entered criticality before the pressure led to the bursting of its confinement, spreading a large volume of radioactive elements in the surrounding area.

Immediate stoppage was required and Života, first on the scene, shutdown the reactor. Simultaneously, Dangubić submerged the neuron rods in cooling water to initiate an emergency shutdown. Catastrophic meltdown averted. The toxic damage, however, had been done. All researchers had been exposed to a severe dose of radiation[viii].

You may be aware of the consequences of uncontrolled radiation on the human body but it's worth detailing the circumstances at Vinča. First, we need to understand the basic lingo of a nuclear physicist. The measure, Gy, meaning Gray, is defined as the absorption of one joule of radiation energy per kilogram of matter. Its how scientists assess the extremity of exposure. A low dose, up to perhaps 0.35 Gy, will leave you feeling nauseous and with basic flu-like symptoms. At Vinča, the exposure levels were calculated to have been between 2 and 4.4 Gy. With this exposure your blood cells begin to die: your immune response weakens due to a drop in white cell count, uncontrollable bleeding due to a lack of platelets, and anaemia due to a reduction of red blood cells. Within 24 hours, you will show signs of acute radiodermatitis, things like red patches, peeling skin, and sometimes blistering. Higher than 4 Gy and you'll also see vomiting, diarrhoea, dizziness, and fever. Without treatment, you could die within a few weeks.

Exposure to radiation has an impact at cellular level. Recall the image of Rosalind Franklin's DNA. Two strands on the outer edge, weaving like a rollercoaster track, with horizontal rungs connecting between them: a bit like a twisted ladder. It contains all our biological information, the code that makes us who and what we are. Radiation attacks your DNA, splitting the strands apart and, while our body can fix much of the damage, some of it cannot be repaired. In trying, cellular mutations occur which lead to secondary implications of radiation, most notably cancer.

As the reality set in, the team of six were evacuated to the local hospital in Belgrade but, with nuclear knowledge in its infancy, it was clear the local medics had no idea how to treat the patients.

In overall command of the Vinča Nuclear Institute at the time was physicist, Pavle Savić. Instrumental in the creation of the institute, he was at the forefront of Yugoslavia's nuclear advancement during this period. Following a six-month scholarship in France in the late 1930s, Savić worked in partnership with Irène Joliot-Curie on a research project and, faced with six exposed scientists, Savić's historic connection with France was to be the solution.

On 16th October, the day immediately following the incident, the whole group were on a JAT Airways flight to Paris. Their greatest hope of survival rested in the hands of a French immunologist and transplant pioneer based at the Institut Curie.

First human bone marrow transplants

Dr. Georges Mathé, 36 years old at the time, was born in Nièvre, France. He'd earned his medical degree from the University of Paris and fought with the Resistance against the Nazis in World War II. He was slender and balding, always wore a pristine white knee-length laboratory overcoat and each wavy line on his furrowed brow told a story of painstaking study through the microscope.

When the Yugoslav group were wheeled into the Institute they were immediately placed on a course of antibiotics. Their conditions continued to worsen over the coming days and weeks. Their hair had fallen out in huge clumps and they were plagued night and day by bouts of sickness and infections.

The blast had totally wiped out any remnants of immunity. Their bodies simply could not defend themselves from any type of viral attack. At this stage, something as innocuous as a common cold could have wiped them out.

Drastic action was needed if they were to survive. It was now the beginning of November and, with winter approaching, Mathé decided he must try something unorthodox. He devised a plan to replace the destroyed immune system with a healthy graft of extracted blood from voluntary donors. Mathé's research led him to believe that if he could replace with healthy new blood things may improve. This had never been done before in humans and did not come without significant risk.

The call was put out to Parisian blood donors with matching blood types to the patients. Within days, five extraordinary humans walked through the doors of the Institut Curie, on Rue d'Ulm in the 5th Arrondissemont of Paris. With so little known at the time, they assumed full responsibility for any side effects of their blood donation – pain, fatigue, infections and even death. When they arrived at the hospital on the day of the procedure, they could not be certain they would return home.

On November 11, 1958, physicist Radojko Maksić became the first person to receive a bone marrow graft from an unrelated donor[ix]. Mathé had drawn the marrow from a bone in volunteer's lower back, before injecting it into a vein in Maksić's arm. The procedures on the other four Yugoslavs followed and, by 16th November 1958, all irradiated physicists had received grafts.

Mathé wasn't alone in his approach to trialling new procedures, as we'll discover, but pioneering work of this nature wasn't without questionable methodology. The patients were all remarkably relaxed about the process having been misled into thinking they were receiving another routine blood transfusion. Presumably, Mathé believed that the Yugoslavs had nothing to lose.

The days following the transplants were key and, remarkably, five of the six of the physicists began to show clear and considerable signs of recovery. The donor marrow, grafted into the patients, had seemingly been accepted and was circulating the body. This was not the case, however, for our early morning cyclist, Života Vranic. The dose of radiation he'd received, the highest of the group, turned out to be fatal. He became the first human in recorded history to die as a direct result of a nuclear reactor catastrophe[7].

For Mathé and his team, however, they'd opened a new door. Studies in the U.S. the year before had attempted to transplant blood cells into terminally ill patients but, while it didn't kill the patients, it hadn't worked. What's more, they'd used blood cells from foetuses and corpses. There was no telling what impact extracting cells from living donors would have.

Weeks passed and the remaining patients continued to regain health. They were becoming stronger and effects of the radiation subsided day after day. Yet by mid-January 1959, two months after the transplant, Mathé couldn't see any donor cells in their blood flow. They were generating their own healthy blood again which meant the 'grafts' hadn't stayed in the system.

Mathé's new approach had saved lives. The patients had lived and he'd achieved the first ever recorded bone marrow transplant. Fundamentally, though, the procedure was deemed a failure.

A little confusing, right? Well, the white cells of the newly produced blood had gone straight to work, rushing around the body and

---

[7] Despite a much larger radioactive explosion in 1957 at the Kyshtym disaster in the Soviet Union, now known to be the third largest ever incident behind Fukushima and Chernobyl, no confirmed deaths were recorded for some years.

warding off infection. The reprieve meant the faulty blood was eventually flushed from the system, as happens with all blood, and bone marrow was then able to get back to work. Once the initial surge had patched up the problem, foreign blood was slowly kicked out of circulation. In this specific instance, an induced case of immunodeficiency, it did the trick. The problem was that for someone with genetically faulty blood and more chronic longer-term problems with immunity, it would not resolve the issue.

They learned that if bodies receive large doses of radiation, transplanted blood seems to be more easily welcomed. If you want a new immune system to go work, an existing immune system needs to be 'asleep'.

It begged the question, could they build on this? If someone's immune system was entirely shot, could a stranger's blood save their life?

What Mathé achieved at the Institut Curie was a glorious success. One person died but five people's lives were saved due to the quick action, and slight bending of the rules, of a vanguard scientist. His intention to permanently swap out the patients' blood had not worked. Nor was he quite sure *how* the patients had survived. But his boldness paid off. A leap of scientific faith by one of the original innovators.

That nuclear disaster inspired a new approach and Mathé's insight laid the foundation of a global movement that would revolutionise the treatment of blood disease.

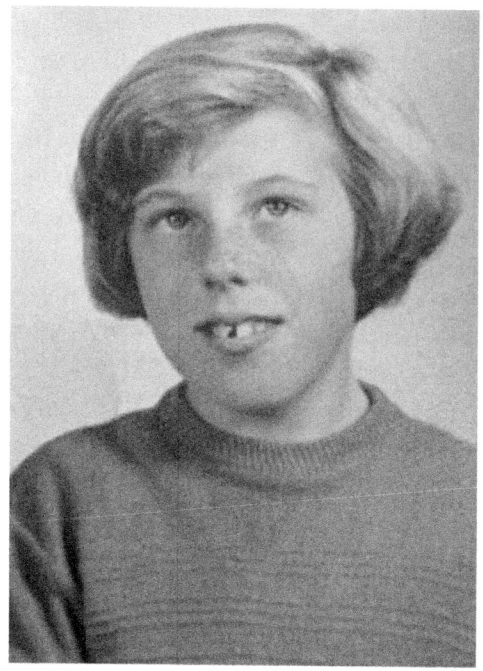

Growing up
1945-1966

As a child, young Elisabeth didn't take kindly to the deep voice of her father. The first time she heard it, at the age of nine-months, her vocal objection to the stranger was loud and relentless. Three-months earlier, in August 1945, WW2 had finally ended but demobbing soldiers was a drawn-out process. Mollie, Elisabeth's mother, deeply wished for her husband Denis to return home from war.

As the atom bomb dropped on Hiroshima, effectively signalling the conclusion, Mollie remembered a specific conversation she'd had in an air-raid shelter in London at the beginning of the Blitz. An elderly gentleman, proud and stoic, stood beside her as bombs detonated above saying, "this is bad enough, but one day they will split the atom and make a destructive weapon that will destroy our world." Quite incredible really, Mollie thought, that as deadly blasts boomed above their heads, he could conjure up a more dreadful set of circumstances. Now it had happened.

It took a time for her little girl to come around. To prevent keeping the rest of the street awake, Mollie would lie holding her daughter's soft hand through the bars of the cot at night for what seemed like an age before she slept. By the time she withdrew her own hand it was cold and numb. They desperately needed to move from this tiny London terrace. Somewhere in the countryside, with space to run and play, where the air was free of city smog. Elisabeth was nearly two years old when, during a snowstorm in the freezing winter of 1947, the family relocated to a cute little house in the Parish of North Mymms, not far from London.

The six years post-war were tough; austerity gripped and everything was in short supply. "I went shopping with a long list", Mollie wrote in her diary at the time, "and all I came back with was a headache and a toilet roll. I shall have to manage somehow to wash Elisabeth's nappies tomorrow without any soap."

Elisabeth was a small, determined and energetic little girl with her long, fair hair, usually seen in two 'pigtails'. She developed a strong maternal instinct early, joyfully wheeling her dolls pram up and down the driveway. Dolls took it in turns to be pushed along with her two white rabbit toys, Timmy and Snowy.

Surrounded by open country, Elisabeth and her friends enjoyed the freedom of nature as they grew up. They didn't know the violence of war. Elisabeth was boisterous and agile, climbing trees to the topmost branch long before her friends, always ensuring they were aware of the fact. She was a risk taker, frequently venturing to 'The Ditch', a frightening spot in the woods where imaginative games played out. Bizarre objects floated in this shallow, murky strip of water where two fields joined. One discovery was a dead ginger cat bobbing ominously on the surface, drifting in their direction. They ran home as fast as their legs would carry them. The Ditch held a dark mystery for the children.

Elisabeth became more self-willed through her school years, a born rebel with a quick temper. But she never sulked or bore resentment. She had an inborn integrity and could always be trusted to tell the truth. She continued to take risks. Her lithe figure gracefully executing non-stop cartwheels on golden sands, riding her bicycle, skating on the ice-rink or coaxing her horse into a gallop. She was always at her happiest when active.

Perhaps being so venturesome led Elisabeth to her fair share of mishaps. She returned home from school one day clutching tightly half of her newly grown front tooth. "Can you stick this on for me, Mummy? I fell off the climbing frame." She had to wait until she reached her teens before her rather large and protruding front tooth, sliced down the centre, could be capped. Then she had to wear a brace to correct the prominence.

As for the rest of her appearance, her grey/blue eyes were long and expressive under brows that resembled the soft touch of a bird's wing with their delicate, upward sweep. She considered her nose to be too high-bridged and would have gladly exchanged it for a smaller, pert model, but she was told it lent character to her face. Her smile had a radiance that transformed and her character possessed magnetism and vitality.

In her teens, Elisabeth developed acne. It was a sore trial, all concoctions and remedies prescribed by dermatologists were to no avail. She hated her appearance but rejected covering with make-up, it was far too painful to apply. Tests revealed a curious cause; her white blood cell count was low, a weakened immune system, she was told. It simply meant her body struggled to fight off bacteria and infection as easily as the rest of her friends. Not a big deal, in the grand scheme of things, but mortifying for a teenage girl. For a significant time, Elisabeth withdrew from a normal social life. Hiding coincided with the family moving house, away from her friends to a far-off London suburb. Elisabeth drifted into a depression, her confidence evaporated, and she suffered immensely from enforced solitude. Medication was prescribed and the local doctor explained to Mollie, "as long as she doesn't come under too much stress her illness won't return. She is vulnerable and has had an emotional illness."

In a fashion that would become typical of Elisabeth's character in adulthood she took matters into her own hands. All at once she upped and moved back home to North Mymms without her parents, sleeping in spare rooms and on sofas of close friends before securing a receptionist job at the local Veterinary College Field Station. She was just 16 but the move had a positive impact. Her skin was still prone to breakouts, but the tide began to turn and pretty soon she was back in her zone, determined to pack her remaining teenage years full of fun. For Elisabeth, this consisted of dances, parties and boyfriends.

A year later – perhaps realising their departure had done more harm than good - her parents re-joined her back in the place they all knew as 'home'. Mollie couldn't help but feel responsible for causing such troubles during that year separated from her friends. They were relatively laid-back parents, and still trying to make amends, the pair decided to head into London for a meal one evening to allow Elisabeth to host a party at the house. Mollie and Denis stayed out as long as they feasibly could but, when they returned home at midnight, the lights still flashed and they could hear muffled music from their living room. The couple entered to a scene from a movie: teenagers, arms aloft and full of carefree joy, wore smiles as wide as you'd imagine, rocking and rolling to "I Want to Hold Your Hand" by the Beatles. Mollie and Denis were drawn in, dancing with the teenagers in the circle until the final euphoric note faded out and the record clicked to a halt.

Alongside the highs, Elisabeth found herself swallowed up by negative emotions. Doctors didn't have a great handle on mental health at the time, many still using electric shock therapy to 'treat' depression. Elisabeth was 16 when she spent her first summer term at the institute in Somerset. Mark Manor was a residential therapeutic centre for children, an escape from the day-to-day, surrounded by calming countryside and nature. She spent her time mucking out the horses, walking the grounds and speaking with staff (probably trained psychiatrists) about what caused her low mood. These places were whispered about in the 1960s, not at all common knowledge and somewhat frowned upon. Parents would need to think their child particularly disturbed to even consider it. Elisabeth spent a second term at Mark Manor before returning to 'normal life'. Those months would never be spoken of again in the family.

Happy late-teen years followed back home in Elisabeth's Hertfordshire sanctuary. Her chosen work offered great satisfaction; the proximity to needy animals a glimpse into the career she still harboured hopes for. Watching from behind the reception desk she believed she could be a brilliant veterinarian someday but, struggling with the science, she was discouraged. When her 21st birthday came around, Mollie and Denis bought Elisabeth a car. The little red

Renault became her pride and joy. She would be seen everywhere in it. It gave her the freedom to go on day trips with her friends and attend parties without relying on her parents for a ride[x].

It was at a party, later that year, that she met a friendly young boy, Roger. She introduced herself as 'Liz' and fell for him the moment she saw him. His calm and phlegmatic approach the perfect complement to her personality. She continued to enjoy her receptionist job but weekends became the highlight in her life. Roger lived in Cambridge but their lengthy telephone calls during the week were bookended by their Saturdays. When the tall, fresh faced, curly-haired young man arrived at the doorstep, her happiness was complete.

Early courting was a joy; the pair revelled in each other's presence. A year of love passed in a heartbeat. Having lunch one sunny Sunday afternoon, at their favourite Inn in the village, Roger had been acting a little awkward. Not necessarily unusual, Liz thought. They'd just been given their order of ice-cream when he unexpectedly announced he was going to quit smoking, cold turkey.

"Oh, OK. And why is that?"

"Well, I'm saving up to get married." He smiled with his eyes.

Liz's stomach fizzed with delight.

'Thy bone is marrowless'
1972

"Get away from my baby. Don't you dare, we don't need you here." Arms flailing, eyes streaming, voices high-volumed and shrill. Nurses and doctors on the Gomer Berry Ward spun instantaneously to pinpoint the source of unrefined hysteria echoing around the otherwise restful area. It was early afternoon on a Thursday; lunch containers, many hardly touched, had just been collected and a round of bloods taken from those young patients being monitored. Beyond the rows of creaky iron-framed beds, each self-contained in sectioned cubicles, a mother fretted, her face drenched in tears and fear. Her manner was agitated, frenetic grabs aimed directly at the approaching Chaplain, employed by the hospital to administer last rites and comfort the dying.

She wasn't ready to say goodbye. The Chaplain had it wrong. He shouldn't be here. She'd certainly not intended on having a physical altercation with a man of God that morning but, seeing him heading her way, her instinct was to stop him in his tracks. His being here meant only one thing and she wouldn't allow it. Father Morris didn't resist; this reaction was, sadly, common place. He split his time across both Westminster hospital sites, visiting children and adults in their hours of need. He'd come to spend most of his time in Vincent Square and, if he'd permit himself to admit it, most of that time with family members not yet ready to say goodbye.

Pretty soon the mother began to weaken, her iron grip melting under the weight of her dread, and a junior doctor eased her aside, propping up beneath the arms, as Father Morris approached the little girl behind the plastic sheet.

Annette

The child looked weak and desperate. Her eyes met those of the Chaplain and explained, in an instant, that she was forlorn and scared. He was here to prepare her for what was next. Too young to understand the nuance of religion, perhaps a blessing in itself, the purity of youth allowed Father Morris to witness fear in an innocent and virtuous way. This child was exhausted, the cavalry of blood disease demons attacking the fortress of her body were in the final throes, already securely behind enemy lines and picking off the final valiant defenders uniting solemnly in their last stand.

Since her bone marrow transplant four weeks prior, four-year-old Annette had experienced the depths of existence. From her static lying position on a plastic-covered mattress she observed upwards as the emulsion peeled away from the ceiling, sometimes from the corners, other times directly overhead. It was all she could do to distract from how her body was reacting. She'd been born with a malfunctioning immune system, a diagnosis that would unquestionably cause her death without intervention. A bone marrow transplant was her only hope but recovery wasn't going well. It had started when she struggled to swallow, her mouth becoming increasingly dry and sore, raw and inflamed, cracking at the edges like the paint above. It hurt too much to speak, her mouth could barely even open; eating and drinking became almost impossible. Mucositis, a common effect of chemotherapy and radiotherapy, is what the doctors told her mother. What they also knew is that

Annette's gut looked the same inside her body, horrifically damaged from devastating radiation poisoning – like that resulting from a nuclear accident such as Vinca – but this time intentionally carried out by those treating her. The results were devastating. Some days would see litres of diarrhoea flow uncontrollably from her small body, her abdominals writhed in pain, her psyche cried in anguish; both only partially and temporarily eased by opiates.

The family could do nothing but watch on in disbelief. As did the medical team whose decision it had been to choose this last-ditch treatment. A decision to push this child to her absolute limits. To actively try to all but kill her, obliterate the body - and almost the soul - only to rescue, bring it back to life. For a high proportion of the infant patients the results would be catastrophic. Their deaths a disastrous drama, playing out in slow-motion over several weeks, those responsible watching on from the front-row, intent on seeing if the manuscript they wrote was a theatrical extravaganza or a desperate Shakespearean tragedy. Most would reach their end like Annette was now reaching hers. Shrunken and battered, fading on the outside and expiring within.

As Father Morris rested carefully to whisper his final well-practised assurances, lines that only he and Annette could hear, the Professor accountable for her treatment watched on discreetly through the glass.

John Raymond 'Jack' Hobbs

Jack permitted himself a moment of private grief. His efforts hadn't worked. He'd made the decision to put this child through an arduous ordeal, as he'd done with many others before her. Fundamentally, it had failed. While his science was sound, and the merits of his choices thorough, he carried the guilt of losing a life heavy on his heart. Each morning before leaving for work he'd kiss the foreheads of his two little daughters as they ate their breakfast. Their blood was strong, they were perfectly healthy girls. He knew he wouldn't cope to see them suffer, as Annette had. Jack considered his profession a thankless task sometimes, an insurmountable challenge; emotionally taxing with an ability to deflate your faith. He chose to shield colleagues from these moments. He needed instead to remain a leading visionary; someone they saw believing wholeheartedly in the transformative impact their field could make.

John Raymond Hobbs, known as 'Jack', felt he'd already given the outside world a glimpse of why he believed in this treatment. Hobbs was immensely proud to be a physician. He wore a crisp white shirt every day; his navy necktie would prominently display the crest of his place of study. His dark-grey suit, crisp and perfectly fitted, oozed class and professionalism. Clean-shaven always, it was rare to see Jack smile on the job; the close-to squinting sharp focus of his eyes often coming across as a scowl. He didn't have time for anyone unwilling to get up to speed. Jack was a *name* in the world of blood disease.

By now, a few years into his tenure at the Westminster Children's Hospital focused on chemical pathology, Jack's work revolved around the biochemical investigation of bodily fluids such as blood, urine and cerebrospinal fluid. He joined the bone marrow transplantation team at a pivotal time. Another expert in this field, Robert Good over at the University of Minnesota, had recently performed the first successful bone marrow transplant for a severe immunodeficiency disease in 1968 – the first triumph of its kind anywhere in the world. It reignited Jack's energy in the possible. Seeing new and successful treatments was something they could learn from, emulate, and develop further.

Hobbs was an expert, almost unchallenged, when it came to the immune system and immune paresis (which is the full or partial shutdown of a body's defence system), be that congenital (at birth) or acquired. He was someone that thrashed out multiple new theories and concepts each day. New ways to beat the complex and devious circulatory system killing children at a rate of knots. The concept he was betting his professional credibility on, and the lives of children like Annette, was that of bone marrow transplantation.

Last chance saloon

Art and literature through the ages has often alluded to the importance of marrow as the sheer essence of life; rich and nutritious as a food source, possessing warmth, energy, and inner heat, as well as being the seat of vitality. The Greek playwright Euripides (480–406 BC) noted: "Love must not touch the marrow of the soul. Our affections must be breakable chains that we can cast them off or tighten them." Even referenced in Shakespeare's Macbeth: "Avaunt! And quit my sight! Let the earth hide thee! Thy bone is marrowless. Thy blood is cold; thou hast no speculation in those eyes which thou dost glare with."[8].

Jack Hobbs was desperate to put the essence of life back into the marrow. For those in need, it was a last chance saloon.

Two-years prior, back in November 1970, a three-month old baby was admitted to the Westminster Children's Hospital under his watch suffering with severe malaise, loose bowels, anorexia and septic lesions of the skin. Her issues were different to Annette's; immune deficiencies are hugely varied and manifest in unique ways

---

[8] https://www.ncbi.nlm.nih.gov/pmc/articles/PMC3069519/

depending on the person. This little girl suffered with abscesses on her scalp and face, ulceration of the tongue and progressively worsening diarrhoea. After developing a chest infection, she lost 2kg of weight, was no longer able to be orally fed and needed a constant supply of nutrients through a tube. By the New Year, she was alive only by intravenous feeding and incredibly devoted nursing.

Jack Hobbs and the team thought it was caused by severe immunodeficiency. Essentially, her leucocytes – the white blood cells fighting off infection – were not doing their job. Like most diagnoses in haematology, tests suggested something with an unnecessarily complex name: *lymphopenia hypogammaglobulinemia,* and an unacceptably subnormal lymphocyte response. He introduced a protein to stimulate cell division and it showed multiple malfunctions in her blood. It was clear that the little girl was extremely close to death. And she was, indeed, a tiny girl; her affliction leaving her malnourished and gaunt.

Tests of all family members found that her four-year old brother happened to have matching blood, the exact thing they needed to give her a fighting chance. Grafting from a sibling is a calculated risk. There are two types of bone marrow transplant. The first is an autologous[9] transplant which involves the use of the cells of the patient themselves. The second, riskier and less understood, is the allogeneic transplant where physicians would use the blood of a donor.[xi]

It meant using a brand-new (somewhat brutal) method devised in the hospital's lab; they inserted a needle deep into the little boy's hip

---

[9] A useful guide when reading this book. When you read 'auto' before a word, like '<u>auto</u>immune', it means the body's own cells. When a word is prefaced with 'allo', such as '<u>allo</u>geneic transplant', that refers to cells from another being of the same species.

bone to extract 12.5ml of bone marrow and tried to save his sister's life.

A week after the transplant there were a few minor signs of improvement. The diarrhoea became less frequent and her stools became semi-formed. Soon thereafter she was able to take food orally again, her skin lesions began to heal, and the respiratory symptoms reduced significantly. Over the following months, still under observation at the Westminster Children's Hospital, she gained consistent weight and was soon given the green light to return home by July 1971.

It was Jack's first proof. His process *could* work. His department was facing increasing pressure, internally and publicly. With little to no dent in the infant mortality rates, he'd been told it was only a matter of time before funding for this unsubstantiated bone marrow treatment stopped. His bosses continued to back him but, without results, the whole unit would be shutdown. Time was not on his side.

Blood is thicker than water

You may think that we share almost identical blood with our close family members but that isn't strictly true. Each of us has a unique immune system developed in the thousands of years that humans have walked the earth. It's an extremely powerful network able to identify the 'self' and the 'non-self'; to pinpoint when something foreign enters our system and attack it. These foreign cells are called 'antigens', from the French antigène – quite literally, 'not our gene'. If your immune system isn't functioning well, no longer able to distinguish safe and unsafe cells, you'll need to replace it. The closer matched the new surveillance system to your original, the better it will fit in and work in its new surroundings. We inherit all our genetics from our parents, with 50% from our mother and 50% from our father, so we're always only half-matched with either parent when it comes to our chromosomes. Scientists however found that one in every four siblings, with the same parents, have an extremely close genetic match which led to the first sibling bone marrow transplants.

By sheer chance, this sibling was a match. What Jack achieved in this instance was the first unfractionated bone marrow sibling graft for severe primary immunodeficiency. An infant, almost certain to die before her first birthday, was successfully sent home with her family and continued to improve. It was the tonic Jack had needed. A calculated risk, a worrisome gamble, but one he took to preserve a life through ground-breaking new methods. He was starting to justify the hospital's faith in him.

To prove his procedure a success, Jack referred to Greek mythology and a monstrous fire-breathing hybrid creature, composed of the parts of more than one animal.

Chimera, the offspring of serpent-giant Typhon and half-woman, half-snake Echidna, features in Homer's epic poem, Illiad, from the 8th century BC. "She was of divine stock, not of men, in the fore part a lion, in the hinder a serpent, and in the midst a goat, breathing forth in terrible wise the might of blazing fire." A mythical beast comprised of various animal components, all of which are identifiable.

Chimerism, as it became termed in medicine, refers to two or more genetically distinct cell populations derived from more than one individual. In humans, or animals, a 'chimera' is a creature that contains two different sets of DNA.

Looking to determine the success of his unfractionated bone marrow sibling graft, Jack searched the young girl's veins for signs that her brother was in there. Of course, he could see that her health was improving but he needed to find out if the transplant had the intended outcome, if they were really onto something. Taking samples of peripheral blood – the blood that circulates our body – Jack and the team identified male chromosomes in the blood cells in the months following the transplant. That is to say that her brother's blood was being made and circulated, to a substantial degree, inside the little girl's body. Unlike the scientists from the Vinca nuclear accident, this offered convincing proof that the transplant had been a success. Essentially, this young girl now had male blood. She could be categorised as a chimera and became one of the earliest success stories for the bone marrow transplantation team at the Westminster Children's Hospital.

It had been, however, a one-off.

On to the next one

Leaning against the wooden ledge and observing Annette's final hours through the glass, Jack's morale troughed again. This time it hadn't worked, another failure. He turned his back on the little girl, now sleeping, and walked away down the corridor towards his laboratory. He doubted he'd see her alive again. He compartmentalised and refocused on the possible, the next child he'd been tasked with saving, lying just a few beds away from little Annette.

This young boy was just over two-years old and posed a somewhat new challenge to Jack. He had an extremely rare and quite different immune deficiency called Chronic Granulomatous Disease (CGD); a granuloma is a cluster of white blood cells and tissue which, when defective, leave someone incapable of fighting even the most common bacterial infections. Jack Hobbs had been in increasingly close cahoots with his colleague, Dr David James; a blood specialist putting a lot of time and energy into understanding this new specialism of matching patients based on Human Leukocyte Antigens (HLA) – the proteins found on the outside of our cells that fight viruses. It was all very new, only really discovered a few years earlier, but researchers had termed the field, 'tissue typing'. He'd checked all the young boy's family, including his newly born baby brother, but none of them were matches. For Jack, and Dr James, this left only one option. To try something that had never been achieved before. An allogeneic bone marrow transplant; to fill the boy with the bone marrow of an unrelated person with a very similar HLA type.

As things stood, the boy's diagnosis was a death sentence. Surely it was a risk worth taking.

Through a peer in Holland, Jack had already moved things along. A sample from a possible blood match was on its way to London. This new case could be a world first. Little Andrew could go down in history and Jack's dream of transplanting the blood cells of a stranger could be realised.

As he strode, he sharpened his resolve. He'd need super blood cells, those recently found to replicate at scale, to flood their new system and adapt to what the body needed. If he could guide those miniscule cells to sync and reproduce in their new environment, he could change the game.

Finding the source of all life
1963

With the orange glow of morning sunlight warming his face, Ernest fidgeted on his stool and removed his glasses. It was Sunday; he felt the need to work this Sunday. From the window of his top-floor laboratory he observed the bustle down below; members of the congregation made their weekly pilgrimage to the church across the street, young families with dogs traipsed to the nearby park. It was often this way on a Sunday, busier than many other neighbourhoods in the Downtown area.

Ernest always felt a sense of private knowing. Those walking directly by rushed about their weekend routine, awash with blissful obliviousness, no concept of what took place inside the walls of 500 Sherbourne Street. To sustain the mundane, he surmised, the entire reason he was here in the first place.

Returning the mouse to the cage Ernest stepped away from the desk. His workspace was, to him, a splendid array of creation and innovation, numerous experiments unfolding simultaneously in real-time all around him. To an untrained observer it was more of a chaotic assortment of glass jars, test tubes, beakers and Parafilm tape spread across cluttered shelves and tables with no concern for order. But Ernest was methodical, particular and on to something big.

Repositioning his spectacles, he examined the next test subject, and then the next. He was satisfied. Hands a little clammy and heart pounding, Ernest scratched pencil marks onto graphs and added notes to the margins. His typewriter clacked ink onto paper, an audible enforcement of historic record, each punch echoing due reverence.

Jim rounded the corner of the seventh-floor corridor headed towards his lab the following morning, around 07:20am. His momentary early solitude was abruptly disrupted. Striding towards him, paper held aloft and flapping in his right hand, Ernest McCulloch yelled excitedly in his scientific partner's direction.

When they came together, Ernest took a breathy moment to compose. "You gotta see this", he insisted. Jim took the graphed paper; there's only one thing this could be about. A momentary glance at the linear line of crosses was all he required; a reassuring clasp on the shoulder of his partner, Jim initiated their progression back towards the office. "I think today calls for strong coffee".

Stumbling into science

One-half of this scientific duo, Jim Till, was born the second son to a farming father and teaching mother deep in the Great Depression of the 1930s that impacted Canada as severely as anywhere in the world. A third of the population became unemployed and national income plummeted by almost half. Ordinarily quite self-sufficient living off short-horn cattle livestock and crops of their farm, the depression miserably coincided with a harsh drought on the prairies of Alberta and Saskatchewan. The Till family, at one lowly point, were reduced to their last quarter dollar choosing to invest in a pack of matches in the hope their fortunes would change.

Perhaps not an obvious beginning for the person who'd prove the source of all living things. Home life in Lloydminster was basic but happy; hard-up but intellectually alive. Education was important and the brothers, four years apart, attended the only school in town before both heading to university. Jim, the younger, pursued physics by chance; with no great scientific passion but zeal for a challenge, he received a scholarship of $50 to pursue a degree in physics at the University of Saskatchewan.

Somewhat to his surprise, Jim did pretty well, excelling at his scientific studies and the scholarships kept coming. He went on to collect his master's degree and, when an opportunity came up at Yale University, he received another one-year scholarship, this time worth $1,800, from the Canadian Cancer Society to secure his PhD. He was now a certified biophysicist.

Jim had found himself championed at the various institutions in the 1950s by two scientists: Harold Johns and Ernest Pollard. In his postdoctoral year, Till was approached by Johns and offered an exciting job out east at the newly established Ontario Cancer Institute in Toronto, which he gladly accepted. The institute not quite ready so he spent a post-doctoral year on placement at Connaught Farm, a base of laboratories just outside Toronto, working with Drs Gordon Whitmore and Louis Siminovitch investigating cell culture.

It would prove to be a pivotal interlude.

Starting his position in the physics division in 1957, there was a buzz about the place; the Ontario Cancer Institute - or the OCI as staff called it - wasn't to receive patients until the following year affording the team time to get their research and treatment capabilities in place.

The facilities were run, together with Harold Johns, by an eminent histologist called Arthur Ham. Histology is the study under the microscope of the cellular components of tissues that make up our bodies. Ham was a foremost expert in the field and his later publication, simply titled *Histology*, was a staple textbook on shelves in student dorms for decades to come. Despite an ability to transform the most mundane topics into intriguing stories[10], Ham was a reclusive character, rarely seen by colleagues outside the institute on Sherbourne Street. He didn't much like to go out, so instead, invited people to him.

Each week, eager to promote cross-disciplinary cooperation, Ham would host private soirees in the basement where he'd invite all staff to attend. These underground sessions, somewhat resembling the intellectual assemblies of London Coffeehouses of the 17th century, took place in the early evening and allowed staff to become acquainted with one another's professional interests and progress updates in an environment that wasn't so sterile. The room was spacious, if quite chilly, dimly lit with lamps dotted all around. It felt welcoming, a hum of conversation greeted newcomers at the door and there were no chairs; seating considered unconducive to fast-paced discussion. Each session saw different researchers introduce themselves, what they were working on and what ignited fire in their belly. The talks were soon a staple social event in a professional's week at the OCI.

At one such event in June, a man stepped into the central *speakers circle* and began speaking passionately about his latest research project. Confident and animated, his address focused specifically, and expertly, on bone marrow transplants and cell culture. Jim,

---

[10] He also balanced his scientific studies with a passion for tennis, playing on the Canadian Davis Cup team

who'd just spent a post-doctoral year examining this very topic, found the talk particularly interesting. That was the first time he really encountered Ernest McCulloch. A few months later, hearing he was looking for a someone to support his work, Jim remembered the talk and put himself forward.

To the untrained eye the pair were something of an unlikely duo. Ernest was short, almost entirely bald, carried a little extra weight and wore thick-set black-rimmed glasses at all times. Jim towered above his partner at well over six feet, had a full head of thick, wavy dark hair and carried an air of Hollywood style about him. Their backgrounds, too, couldn't have been more different. McCulloch the product of a wealthy family, elite schooling and very early had a career path in science laid out before him. Till, as we know, was a country boy from a hard-up farm on the prairies who sort of willingly stumbled into science. And they got off to a slightly rocky start.

McCulloch's research focused on observing cells at work in mice; removing cells, irradiating cells, injecting cells. A respected teacher, the experienced haematologist had a piercing gaze, eccentric manner, and zero patience for fools. As Till, five-years the junior, set about measuring the radiation dosage administered to the mice, he made a mistake. Until this point they'd kept to their own part of the agreement, working quite independently. McCulloch's short fuse was well-known but Till braved trepidation and owned up to his mistake. Momentary silence and then, rather than ridiculing the young physicist, the admission cemented a trusting professional friendship. Ernest was, above anything, impressed that the physicist admitted to making a mistake; to being fallible. That bonded their partnership which was, from that point on, collaborative always.

This important Toronto partnership thrived on observing and understanding the smallest structural and functional unit of an organism. Cells of a life-form, regardless of belonging to an oak tree, a blue whale or a rat, are all similar in size; each around one-tenth the width of a human hair and pretty much invisible to the naked eye. Such intricate inspection of microscopic parts, by this point the norm to understanding disease, had required a rethink of the phrase 'as far as the eye can see'.

A tiny world of animalcules

Peering intently through a magnifying lens at a substance sitting atop the glass panel below, British scientist, Robert Hooke, announced in 1665 that within the material he could quite clearly identify distinguishable pores set out in asymmetrical rows. Using a microscope about six inches long with two convex lenses inside he examined specimens under reflected light. In his published work *Micrographia* his keen eye noted that they were somewhat similar to the six-sided sections of a honeycomb in structure (Cellulae), or the devotional space of a monk in the monastery (Cella, in Latin). He believed the individual sections to be perforated and porous, with thin walls or film partitions, and labelled each section as a box, or a 'cell'.

Termed as such for the first time, Hooke plunged headlong through the lens deep into a new dimension; an as yet unexplored minuscule cellular world.

This exploration was made possible through the development of the device just mentioned, a microscope, capable of uncovering hitherto unimagined marvels. The first was designed by Galileo Galilei at the turn of the 17th century. More fine tuning with lenses was done by Dutch spectacle makers, Janssen and Lipperhey, who realised that by placing different types and sizes of lens in opposite ends of tubes they could make objects appear much larger than they actually were.

And they were not the only ones in their country discovering the power of reflective glass.

In the thriving city of Delft in the Dutch Republic, the same year that Hooke's *Micrographia* was published, a cloth merchant purchased an understated property on the Hippolytusbuurt, right on the canal in the boutique district, with dreams to transform it into a profitable drapery business. At the time Delft was the fourth largest city in the country with a newly bustling economy benefitting, due to its proximity to a thriving port, from foreign trade: cotton, tobacco and sugar from the West Indies; textiles, spices and other goods from India.

As exotically elegant new fabrics, delicate lace and fine cloth arrived in the city each week, draper Antoine van Leeuwenhoek, found himself needing to inspect more closely the quality of the thread presented to him. Relatively new to the scene, he was perhaps singled-out by the more seasoned tradesmen as an easy mark. A shake of hands on a recent deal had caught him out. Instead of the fine silk and quality linen he'd been assured of, later inspection found these fabrics to be lacking in excellence, substandard in every way to the aspiring draper.

Antoine was adamant that no more merchants would catch him out. He needed to get a closer look as soon as they left the ship; to inspect the intricacies of the thread, observe the quality of the yarn, identify any minor fallibilities of the fabric. Existing lenses readily available at the time were primitive, falling far short of his needs, so he took it upon himself to experiment with lens making, each time finding methods to further magnify the material underneath.

As it turned out, his technique – focused on adjusting untainted, high-quality glass spheres - went far beyond the magnifications achieved by anyone else thus far and, soon enough, his inspections too went beyond cloth and lace.

Initially looking at mould, bees and lice, van Leeuwenhoek went on to inspect wood, plants, fish and insects, all the while documenting his findings in letters addressed to the Royal Society in London. The tiniest slice of bark or slither of a fish caught in the estuary revealed so much movement, so much life. He was reluctant to publish his findings at first; after all, he was just a businessman with no scientific credentials but, encouraged by a physician friend, continued prolifically submitting his observations until, in 1673, his work was eventually published in the Society's journal.

So many letters of notable discovery were being written, and sketched, by van Leeuwenhoek that the editor of the Royal Society, Henry Oldenburg, learned Dutch in order to make accurate translations. It was when observing rainwater under the microscope that Antoine used the term 'animalcules' to describe the tiny animal-like beasties he could see moving through his lens and, on close inspection of his own teeth, reported miniscule single-cell creatures alive and moving; the prospect of which was previously entirely unknown. While Hooke discovered what he called a 'cell', van Leeuwenhoek became the first person in history to observe a *living cell*. Using his unique method of microscopy, and a curiosity for the natural world, this cloth merchant became the 'Father of Microbiology' with the creation of microscopes that could magnify up to 500 times. This led to his discoveries including bacteria, muscle fibres, sperm cells and red blood cells.

In total van Leeuwenhoek wrote 190 letters to the Royal Society, all remain with the Society's library and are accompanied by illustrations of what he'd seen, and by the time of his death was their most published author, by far. He was visited by Kings, Queens and aristocrats all desperate for a glimpse into his new kingdom of tiny creatures; ferocious leaders from William of Orange and Queen Mary II, to Tsar Peter the Great.

The importance of van Leeuwenhoek's microscopes (of which there were around 25) and his discoveries influence and energise us to this day. Not only do we now regularly brush our teeth, understanding the harm of bacteria (or animalcules), but the ability to inspect cells under a powerful magnifying lens has revolutionised modern medicine. What's more in 1687, a relentlessly curious van Leeuwenhoek began playing around with the simple coffee bean. He roasted the bean, cut it into slices and spied up-close its spongy interior. When he pressed the bean, an oil oozed out so he boiled it with rainwater twice and set aside the world's first cup of coffee. Goodness knows his surprise when he came to tasting his concoction, or if Till and McCulloch recognised the link as they caffeinated their way through their own excitable discovery almost three centuries later.

The microscope continued to be developed over the next few hundred years; lenses became more powerful and glass spheres purer, allowing scientists and scholars to study the mystical world through the eye piece. Until this point no one understood what caused disease and illness. Theories existed, and many claimed to have remedies and cures, but it was the ability to see agents of disease, visible for the first time that allowed experts to identify, name and prevent diseases.

How do cells actually work?

Regardless of extensive research very little was truly understood of the potential of 'cells'. Exactly what each did, or indeed where they came from, was still unknown. That was until the mid-1800s when a huge scientific fight broke out in Bavaria that would kickstart our knowledge of cell theory.

Prussian-born neurologist Robert Remak, from Posen (now

Poznań, Poland), was the son of humble tobacconists but had enrolled at the University of Berlin after being declared a Prussian citizen. At the time of his greatest discovery, he was a relatively unknown name in cell theory circles and, due to the following circumstance, has remained so ever since.

Working quietly on experiments into nerve tissue at the Charité Hospital, Berlin, he published his research to little or no acclaim. It hadn't been a straightforward journey to this point; barred from teaching by Prussian law, which closed that profession to Jews, he continued his research as an unpaid assistant in a laboratory and supported himself by private medical practice. By 1847 Remak had a considerable quantity of work under his belt and, as a consequence, secured a lectureship at the University of Berlin becoming the first Jew to hold such a role; so momentous an achievement that the newspapers made a splash of the appointment. Remak had followed the centuries-old debate in scientific quarters regarding the theory of spontaneous generation; the belief that living species can arise, not necessarily a descendent from organisms like themselves but, in fact, from non-living matter. For example, at the time people believed that a wriggling grumble of maggots were produced by rotting meat or that a patch of wet soil gave life to amphibians, such as frogs and toads. Even famous Greek thinker, Aristotle, subscribed to the idea that life could be created by non-living material, if that material contained pneuma ("vital heat"). Remak was motivated by the recent proposals of French scientist, Bartholomew Dumortier, who used the phrase 'binary fission' for the first time stating that cells divide to create new versions of themselves and allow plants to grow. According to Dumortier, a mid-line partition would emerge, connecting the original cell to a brand-new cell and he claimed that it "seems to us to provide a perfectly clear explanation of the origin and development of cells, which has hitherto remained unexplained".

As part of his own research Remak had been closely observing the red blood cells from chicken embryos under the microscope as they progressed through the various stages of development and had witnessed similar such inexplicable divisions himself. Convinced his eyes had not deceived him, Remak was adamant that the established spontaneous generation theory was incorrect. He published his papers boldly stating that, instead, cells copy themselves by dividing and reproducing.

It was a brand-new concept but went ignored for more than three years until a former junior colleague at the Charité Hospital, Rudolf Virchow, decided that he may be onto something. Rather than promote already published papers, however, Virchow (a much more socially known figure in pathology circles) plagiarised the findings, portraying them as his own. In Latin he stated, 'Omnis cellula e cellula', which translated to 'all cells arise only from pre-existing cells.' It got a bit ugly and a very public war of words broke out between Virchow and Remak, the latter never really receiving the credit he deserved for a pivotal discovery in the timeline of cell theory.

Virchow wasn't all bad, though. An eminent figure in his field he had, just a few years earlier in 1847, independently observed abnormal increases in white blood cells in some of his patients, correctly identifying the condition as a blood disease. He named it leukämie; later Anglicised to leukaemia[xii].

Cells were now known to be the building blocks of life and believed to be crucial components to all living things on earth. But despite now being visible, their origins, workings and true worth were all still completely out of the grasp of leading global scientists.

As Till and McCulloch reviewed their data on the windy Monday morning in Toronto, the foundations of cell theory, laid out by Remak, wasn't the only predecessor they kept in mind. The controversial work of a Russian embryologist 50 years prior took cell theory onto a new level.

At the dawn of the 20th century, Alexander Maximov transcribed his latest observations: "I have now found that these primitive blood cells (which is what I call them), contrary to what would be commonly expected, are not erythroblasts but completely undifferentiated elements with a round bright nucleus and narrow basophilic cytoplasm. These are neither red nor white blood corpuscles."

A very peculiar claim from the esteemed scientist; that the blood cells he was observing were neither red nor white; the only options currently known to science. He further asserted, "...[U]nder the influence of stimulation, they [the cells] can be mobilized and become transformed into free, wandering ... elements ...".

In this paper of 1908, Maximov tabled the term "stem cell" for scientific usage. He demonstrated that all blood cells develop from a common precursor cell; that there's one distinct type of parent blood cell that generates all the offspring cells, both red and white. They were seen to him under the microscope as a clump of cells, perhaps like a colony or, as he described, "an island", from which all other blood cells originated. It had previously proved impossible to identify such a cell and define it in any meaningful way.

In making this leap, Maximov proffered the unitarian theory of haematopoiesis stem cells (the blood forming stem cell), that they could be found in the medulla of the bone (bone marrow) and have the unique ability to give rise to all the different mature blood cell types and tissues.

This is the birth of the stem cell story. Alexander Maximov died suddenly in Chicago on 3rd December 1928, a decade after emigrating to the United States during the Russian Revolution. When he closed his eyes for the final time and his own cells shutdown, Maximov knew that he left behind a sound concept of blood cell reproduction observed in chicks; parent cells producing child cells to carry out the work of blood circulation. His problem was left unsolved, however, and he couldn't have possibly anticipated the future trajectory of the research he had begun; the transformative science it would yield thanks to two pupils of his writing 500 miles east, at 500 Sherbourne Street.

Proving it, once and for all

Jim Till busied himself reviewing the preserved spleens of sacrificed mice currently under histological examination. Like Maximov, the Toronto researchers had primarily focused on the cells in the spleen, as it was known to be a focal point of blood-creation and the lymphatic system responsible for immunity. Stood in his lab coat, side by side with Ernest, the flesh-like bumps were clearly visible to Jim. As his partner liked to explain. "If I see bumps like that then I count them", and the count was perfectly linear to the number of bone marrow cells the mouse had been administered. It appeared that every ten-thousand cells equated to a bump on the spleen. Observable bumps. If these newly formed colonies of cells had derived from that single cell, then this was, indeed, a very big deal.

The research method wasn't pretty. The team blasted their subject mice with destructive doses of radiation, enough to mimic the catastrophic effects of a nuclear bomb or the incident at the Vinča power station. The aim was to completely destroy the immune system, rendering their white blood utterly useless, then introduce new cells to determine if fresh blood can reproduce; this would show if bone marrow transplants can rebuild new blood in animals whose own marrow was destroyed. They used inbred mice[11], with genetically identical cells, so they were confident the transplants would not be seen as foreign and attacked. They hypothesised that 'marrow cells injected intravenously into lethally irradiated animals will permit the survival of a proportion of recipient animals and that the decrease in mortality is a function of the number of cells given'. The more marrow cells introduced, the greater the chance new blood cells would grow and thrive. But something more: when examined, the new colonies contained a mixture of red blood cell precursors alongside white blood cell precursors. A single cell *must* have given rise to the colony which, if true, meant that a single cell must have given rise to different types of blood cells.

This was spectacular. That all types of blood cells could stem from one super cell. A brand-new theory of how blood was made. That this super cell could adapt how it replicated based on what the body needed. It was a stunning theory, now they needed to prove it. To verify unequivocally that all cells in the colony, no matter how dissimilar, derived from a founder. That they were all clones.

They published their extraordinary findings in 1961 with an article in the peer-reviewed *Radiation Research* journal with the title, 'A Direct Measurement of the Radiation Sensitivity of Normal Mouse Bone Marrow Cells'. It wasn't particularly catchy, nor widely read; most scientists were too focused on the recent discovery of DNA to learn more about these 'colonies of proliferating cells'.

There was more work to be done to prove their theory. They carried out test after test after test, introducing bone marrow cells and observing what happened at 100- and 1000-times magnification

---

[11] Inbred mice refer to the brother-sister mating over 40+ generations which leads to almost genetically identical twins. Not a process that can be replicated in humans.

under the microscope. In their words, "The spleen colony procedure may, therefore, be regarded as an in vivo single-cell technique, analogous to the well-known in vitro single-cell experimental systems."

That is to say that a single stem cell would repopulate an entire marrow. All red blood cells, white blood cells and platelets in that circulatory system would originate from a single injected bone marrow cell. Specifically, from a hemopoietic 'stem cell'; a stem cell that can create the whole gambit of blood cells.

They'd discovered a source of life.

In 1963, Jim, Ernest and Andy Becker published an article[xiii] in the popular journal, *Nature*, this time to much greater acclaim. They had the science world's attention and followed it up the same year proving that the spleen colonies could replicate, creating even more new colonies of cells.

The knowledge of stem cells may have been around for some time but this group of Canadian scientists were the first to prove functionality and offer a clear definition. That they must be capable of self-renewal, they must be able to create differentiated descendants and be capable of extensive proliferation.

Before this discovery, bone marrow was seen as somewhat of a 'black box', little known or understood. Beyond the pure science of it all, the potential usefulness of this discovery was quickly apparent. A stem cell was able to replicate in a new environment and have the ability to multiply at scale from just one single super cell.

For people desperate for healthy new blood, perhaps from someone else, this was a pivotal moment.

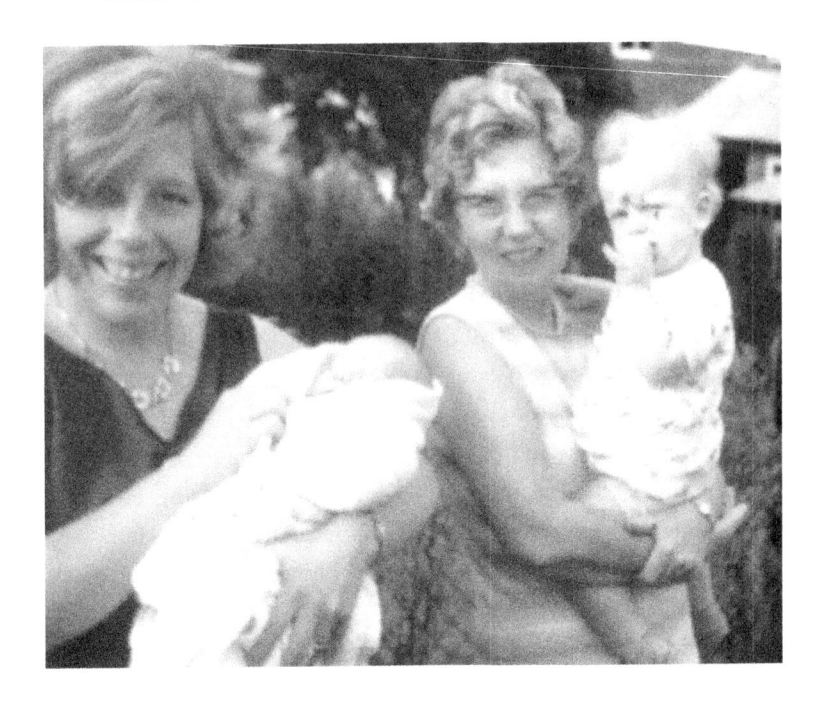

Andrew Bostic
1970-1972

Two white butterflies drift with effortless synchroneity in an English summer scene. Purity of colour differentiating the players from the pallid backdrop; they enter from the wings to grace the static space with mesmeric creativity. The dance begins. Each perfectly aware of the other's moves; each cognisant of their own. Locked into tight, ascending circles in an airy dalliance, landscape is forgotten, briefly, as focus fixates on these aesthetic enthrallers. A flurry of delicate swirls, a crescendo of irrepressible performance; then a parting, a fade, a dissolve stage left, knowing they, or those like them, will appear again.

Liz observed the silent routine in a trance. She felt still and calm, but empty. The intensity of the flit fitting the profundity of her dread.

What remained, when the nurses left the scene, was her son; the single most important thing in her life who, for a few uncontrollable minutes, became a distant blur behind a choreographed flutter of professional performance.

Her boy was sleeping. The needles and body jolts now so common he no longer deemed them worthy of his consciousness. Liz felt guilt for momentarily losing focus but granted herself reprieve; when he's in a dreamworld she can't control his happiness. Even when awake she invariably felt powerless; had for as long as she could remember; her role as mother and protector banished by the evils of disease.

His eyes darted within the confines of sleep, a twitch of the leg and a lick of the bottom lip. In a dream her boy can run and dance and live out the pleasures of his pleasing. A place of endless possibilities and no limitations. Pain cannot harm him in that world. When he falls asleep, where does he go? Sat alone at the foot of the bed, unaccompanied in these early morning hours, she longed for him to remain in that preferable setting. Even monstrous nightmares promised a kinder experience.

Her mind drifted again from the enormity of matters. You can't help but respect the complexity of nature. As a virus attacks, destroys and mutates to evade extinction, so too a cancer meticulously plots its path. A cockroach of a disease, evading a multitude of attacks from the greatest powers the human mind can throw at it. You may think you've got it; smoked it out or crushed it to a paste, overzealous but thorough. Yet soon it appears again, left behind by the last, a symbol of defiance.

She often dwelled on her role in all this. Her own genetics the very reason he lay before her, fighting for his life. To have died on her wedding day would have saved his pain.

*

The pews had been filled in the ancient St Etheldreda church in Hatfield, Hertfordshire, with Mollie, her mother, sat on the front row beaming with excitement. It was four-years ago, 23rd March 1968 – a Saturday – and the guests, most having made the short journey up from London that morning, were beginning to show signs of polite restlessness. A noticeable fidgeting rose while others grew weary of the organist repeating a limited repertoire. The bride was over 30-minutes late.

When Liz finally walked up the aisle, arm in arm with her father, the tension in the room dissipated. A beautiful service played out and only when she turned back to face her loved ones after the proclamation of wedlock that a cut on the bridge of her nose, and splatters of blood on the front of her dress, could be seen.

Just minutes after leaving the house on her very special day Liz's car door had suddenly flung wide open while taking a corner and oncoming car swerved straight into them. Had it not been for her father, Denis, instinctively grabbing her around the waist, she'd have been thrown out and likely ended up under the other vehicle. As it happened her head flew forward under braking where she cracked her nose on the front seat.

Each time she looked back at the bizarre events, she found no new explanation for how such chaos had occurred but what she was certain of was that her dad had saved her life. The car was ruined so a neighbour, still wearing his gardening clothes, sunk his pitchfork in the dirt and hastily drove them to the church. A few quick repairs to her makeup in the backseat and no harm done; she wouldn't allow this to interrupt her wedding day.

Checked over by the on-call doctor, who found no broken bones but warned of shock, Liz set off to the hotel where their reception was taking place. A brandy awaited her arrival; news travelled fast. Downing it she hadn't even notice that the venue had double-booked, leaving her guests to celebrate in a much smaller room adjacent to the banquet hall. Again, this wouldn't ruin the day.

When it was time to leave the celebrations, suffering a little from the effects of delayed shock and brandy, the couple dashed through a vibrant shower of confetti and well-wishers before turning, as they met the getaway vehicle, for a final photograph. The snapshot pauses a moment in time; the gash on her nose and bruising now clearly visible, the blustery wind catching her veil leaving her soft, light-brown hair to frame her face. They were now officially Mr and Mrs Bostic. Dazed but visibly content, she leant into Roger whose arm wrapped around in a protective grasp. 'Bride in Accident on Wedding Day' the local newspaper headlines later read, accompanying this cherished photograph.

That was the moment, she felt, where it could have turned out so differently. Had it ended that day. This being the pivotal pause; as a ball tossed towards the sky gains height, defying forces against it then slows and, for the briefest moment, rests delicately serene in mid-air. To end it here would avert the fall.

Liz watched her youngest child sleeping in front of her. He seemed calm. When confronting these dark recesses, she was invariably thinking of her first-born son.

His name was Andrew.

*

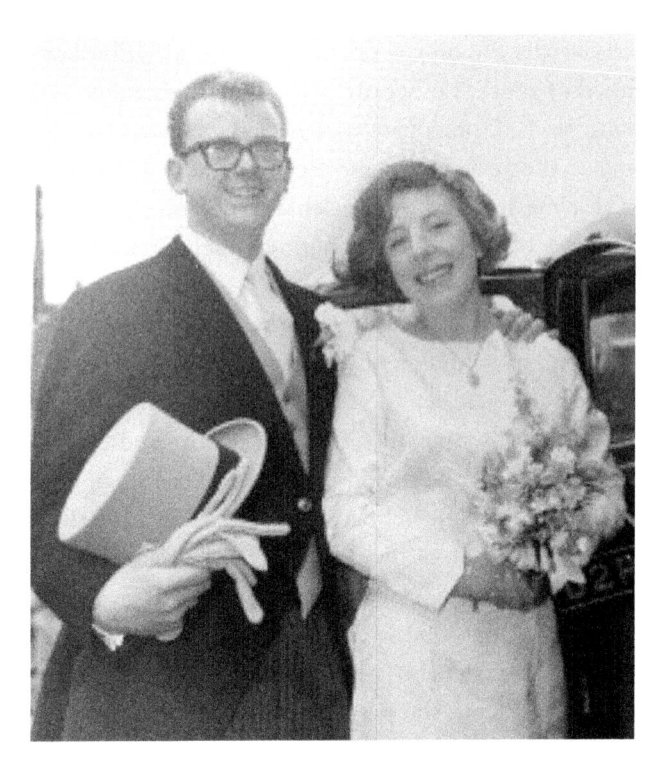

In May, the year following their wedding, Liz discovered that she was pregnant. It hadn't been the plan. They had wished to start a family together and the pair were delighted at the prospect but had hoped to settle into marriage and homelife before venturing into parenthood. Liz sat one evening with her mother to watch the devastating television drama 'Cathy Come Home': the heart wrenching descent of a young couple with children into poverty and homelessness. The believable fiction overwhelmed her with dread; that their life may imitate the art. What if she too couldn't protect her baby? Roger's job at a chocolate factory as a store foreman, and hers as a temp secretary, were fairly steady but you just never know, she would think. They decided to put their best foot forward, securing a beautiful Victorian terrace cottage close to her parents – number 21, Holloways Lane in Welham Green.

Their pink and gold baby, Andrew Bostic, was born on 17th February 1970: a tiny, unwrinkled child with a blush pink face, azure blue eyes and a cap of golden red hair. Liz relayed her joy down the phone to Mollie. "Oh mum, he is so beautifully perfect." The nurses fussed over him straight away, talking quickly and showing no attention to the mother. One very young nurse carried Andrew into a cot next to Liz's bed, leaned over and said a prayer out loud. It seemed a little strange, perhaps ominous, but Liz didn't take too much notice.

Motherhood suited Liz. Her radiant boy thrived, gained weight as expected, slept through the night and very rarely cried. A new mum she revelled in the simple contentment she derived from planning the forthcoming years: she'd have children close together in years, perhaps three in total; when they started school she'd reduce her hours to work part-time, spending longer spells in the home nurturing her family.

By Andrew's first birthday Liz was already pregnant with a second child and she exuded the blissful serenity of a young women of 27 prizing the modest joys her life brought her. Their house was now a home; their jobs fulfilling, extended family close-by, and her sunny-tempered Andrew would breathe pleasure into each day. An only-child herself she'd always wished for a large family. Walking in the local park with her mother one day, she watched Andrew jump blissfully in puddles and feed ducks, a beaming smile reaching across his face. Liz's adoration was boundless. "It's just as well I'm having another one soon', she proclaimed to Mollie, 'or I might spoil him".

At 13-months Andrew's health took a turn when he developed a fever and swollen neck, enough to warrant a visit to the clinic doctor and, the following day, admission to the local hospital. Checks were carried out, and mumps ruled out, but no diagnosis could be made as nurses patted him down with cool, damp cloths to reduce his temperature. Liz saw in the doctors' mannerisms that they were worried and her imagination ran riot. When an abscess developed on one of his glands the surgeons chose to operate and Andrew remained in a small cubicle on the children's ward for more than eight weeks. Each morning Liz would arrive at 7am, heavily pregnant, observing as a team drained one painful abscess only for another angrier one to appear shortly thereafter. No matter how many blood samples they wrestled from little Andrew's arms, the medics remained baffled, confused by the refusal of the illness to follow what they'd learned in the textbooks. Sometimes they had to resort to getting blood from a vein in Andrew's neck, so bruised were the arms and hands.

It was torture for Liz.

Mollie would relieve her daughter regularly, and Roger would turn-up on his lunch break, allowing Liz to preserve energy for her unborn child. She would sit by Andrew's cot endlessly reading nursery rhymes. He loved them; an intense look of concentration as the lines were recited. "Again, nannie" he would say as the last page was turned.

In and out of hospital as the weeks went on, sometimes just for antibiotics, other times for overnight stays. The family couldn't comprehend that no one was able to pinpoint what this lingering issue was. If they couldn't diagnose, how could they even begin to treat it?

As a nurse finished her checks on one occasion, she hurried to see the next child, accidentally leaving Andrew's file in the holder at the end of his bed. Liz grasped her opportunity, completely breaking protocol, and the notes read "suspected Chronic Granulomatous

Disease". Without hesitation she cornered the Ward Sister. "What on earth is this disease? I've never heard of it." After brazenly admonishing Liz for reading the secretive file, the Sister explained that, while they didn't actually think he had it, CGD was a rare type of blood disease that they wanted to check for. To test for this Andrew would need to be transferred for a special blood test at the most advanced unit in the country: the Westminster Children's Hospital in Central London.

'Chronic Granulomatous Disease of Infancy', Liz scribbled down in the back of her diary. She couldn't even pronounce it. What did it mean? What if it was serious?

A few weeks later, Roger went to pick up the test results. It was now May; Liz was eight-months pregnant and, despite the odd cough and his neck covered in small scars from removed abscesses, Andrew was definitely more alert and playful. He'd developed a love for music, in particular the nursery rhymes that played on a constant loop from his mother's old record player. "Another record", he'd say as the needle reached the inner ring, crackled and lifted.

His father sat in a small, rectangular office on the second floor of the Westminster Children's Hospital as Dr Kenneth Hugh-Jones, a local consultant paediatrician in St Albans, pawed through a set of papers across a desk. Roger noted that the doctor's manner was warm, quite matter of fact, but in a fashion that both valued clarity of diagnostic and humanity of parental tenderness.

Himself a father of four, "H-J", as he was called on the ward, is one of the unsung heroes of bone marrow transplantation. A detailed leader of paediatric care, he'd never seek the limelight, preferring to support children and families behind-the-scenes. Hugh-Jones paused frequently and spoke directly to Roger as he informed him that indeed his son *did* have the suspected Chronic Granulomatous Disease which, as a result, left it unlikely his child would survive beyond the age of two years old.

Travelling back to Hertfordshire, Roger made the decision to shield his wife from the stress of this news in the final stages of pregnancy. At least for now, he would tell her just as soon as she'd recovered from childbirth. Until then he would keep it locked away. "Not to worry, dear', he announced, smiling cheerfully walking into the living room. "You've got it as well. Some of your cells can't kill bacteria, so that's where he's got it from."

This was, in fact, partly true.

Liz had a genetic mutation that meant only half of her white blood cells had the enzyme to fight bacteria. It had caused her skin blemishes and frequent sicknesses as a teen. A trying situation but not a particularly life-threatening one to her: more susceptible to catching colds, developing spots and longer recovery times but, on the whole, a weak but capable immune system.

"Oh, thank goodness, and I'm still alive". Liz was utterly relieved. Her genes seemed to be the cause of her son's illness but her relatively good health gave renewed hope that all would be well. The impact of Liz's genetic mutation for male offspring, however, could be fatal. X-linked diseases are caused by a mutation to the X chromosome. Women, with two X chromosomes, compensate for the defect with the other unmutated chromosome. Males inheriting X-linked diseases, and with only one X chromosome, can't counter the fault. Any boy would have a 50-50 chance of getting the disease from the mother and, unbeknownst to the couple at the time, they were about to have another.

Simon Peter Bostic was born on July 2nd, 1971. Roger held his second child close, a fine and healthy boy, wizen eyed and wrinkled like a little old man. Liz took a little persuading. She refused to hold Simon, thinking him the ugliest baby she ever saw. Perhaps intent on not loving this son to protect her own emotions. Perhaps sullen as she'd prayed for a girl. "Come on now, surely you'd like to hold him", the midwife would say. "Take him away, I don't want to touch him", Liz would reply. Despite remaining in the dark as to the full extent of the immunity problem, fear gripped her. She was glad he was so red-faced and wrinkly, it made it easier not to love.

Her reluctance didn't last for long, bending down when no one else was around and cradling her baby. The boys were acquainted at home the following morning; Andrew, too young for jealousy, peering over the crib chattering to his brother in his own way.

Within days a test was set up to check if Simon would also be affected by the disease and, in a few weeks, it was confirmed that yes, he was. The fatality of the prognosis was still unknown to anyone but Roger: he bore the pressure, accompanied every step of the journey but holding weight for everyone. That summer they danced. The couple were still young, just three-years married, and their trials had renewed their zest for life. The ballroom provided a space to lose themselves, their steps synchronised but otherwise increasingly out-of-touch.

The world chilled as November arrived. Both boys suffered worsened health taking it in turns, or sometimes concurrently, to spend time at the local hospital. Simon, just over three-months old, had developed an abscess under his chin, which was drained leaving a scar. Andrew's glands and temperature continued to flare. 'H-J', the consultant paediatrician from St Albans out-patients ward who also worked at the Westminster Children's Hospital, queried why Liz's husband so rarely attended with the boys. "Next time you come, tell him to come too", Hugh-Jones insisted. "I'd like a word with him."

The starting pistol had been fired. Within days Roger and Liz were at the clinic. The Consultant, distracting Liz on an errand to the pharmacy, gave the ultimatum to Roger that now was the time to explain the fate of the children to their mother. No more waiting. She sensed something was wrong on the car journey home and, upon entering their house in Welham Green, he revealed to her everything that he'd been told.

Only now the realisation of circumstance was laid out before them. Despite their outwardly normal appearance, the boys would both die, possibly before they each reached 24-months. The parents would lose their children to an invisible disease; something the medical world did not know enough about to cure. Roger returned to the chocolate factory; unwilling or unable to face his wife's sorrow. Liz muffled her sobs behind closed doors of the terrace.

Attempting to portray a conspiracy of hope, Christmas of 1971 was a joyous celebration. The boys remained healthy, friends popped by frequently, and the Christmas tree which filled the front window heaved with gloriously vibrant decoration and centred their focus. The favourite record player flooded their home with carols and festive cheer, each crackle and click finale met with Andrew's favourite phrase, "another record", and a giggle. The house was awash with gaiety for a brief time. Everyone, except the children, knew this would be their last as a four.

As if what they faced wasn't enough the New Year brought new dread. Suffering a stiff neck, perhaps swollen glands, Roger himself went for a check-up in January 1972 and was prescribed antibiotics. It soon became evident that what they were dealing with, however, was a tumour. Hodgkin's Disease, a rare cancer of the lymph nodes, and plans were made for his treatment: lots of drugs and radiotherapy.

Liz now faced the devastating prospect of losing her entire family. Roger became thin as the treatment drained his body. Without the energy to care for the boys, Liz shouldered additional caring responsibility to keep the men in her life healthy and able to fight invisible demons. Andrew was also becoming frailer by the day. Flinging his arms around his grandparents to hug them on arrival, they could feel his strength depleting. An inflamed spot discovered in the middle of his back, and complaints of tummy ache, led to another visit to the hospital where they were told there was little hope of changing the course of events to follow.

Liz was told she needed to keep the boys free from germs because their bodies were unable to fight infection. She also found out that they could try a procedure called a 'bone marrow transplant'. It meant putting someone else's blood into her child's body. It freaked her out a bit but the hope was that new blood could revamp their immune system. It could fight off infection and keep them alive. The whole family were tested without a moment's hesitation, but no one was suitable. So that was that then. Unless they tried asking outsiders – a feat that had never been achieved before.

On 27th July, Andrew was admitted to the Westminster Children's Hospital with a risky final option on the table. Liz would sit in the little chair next to her son's bed and, as he would sleep, she'd observe the comings and goings of the ward. It was noisy; two rigid rows of metal-framed beds lined long walls, at the end a fully curtained room. That room meant one thing; you'd try to avoid it at all costs. Feet facing inward, children admitted would start in beds at one end and make their way along as their stay extended; beds freed up as other children lay behind the curtains, and then didn't.

A little girl called Wendy sat up in the bed opposite Andrew. She tried to catch his eye by showing him the pages of the comic she was reading. Her favourite was *Judy*, she must have read it front-to-back over 20-times. He showed little interest in her and his ambivalence made both mother's giggle. Shared vulnerability and imperfection. Wendy's mother was as omnipresent as Liz; her father as absent as Roger. Wendy was maybe four years old but looked much older, the rigours of punishing treatment transforming her appearance to that of an elderly lady. Her smooth scalp glistened from the strip light beam above, her hair had long-since deserted her. The skin beneath her eyes drooped and clustered, tired of trying to stay taught, and it veiled sharp cheek bones, protruding as if trying to break the seal. Her skin was now more like a thin layer of film, so delicate that her muscles and tendons were clearly distinguishable. Liz feared the merest touch would rip it open, exposing everything beneath to the glare of the world. Her complexion was entirely beige. Her neck, arms and legs slender and pallid, like a sandy desert gecko. She'd complain of headaches, her nose would bleed uncontrollably, she'd vomit regularly. The body's tedious decline creeps like a vine.

But when she smiled, she really meant it.

All the joy she could muster would transmit across the room, almost physical in its journey and you couldn't help but instantly smile when it reached you. Liz would immediately catch herself, masking the lump in her throat. She couldn't cry at Wendy's helplessness.

One morning, after not touching breakfast, Wendy was wheeled off the ward in her bed and, by the afternoon, her mother whispered news of her death to Liz. Tears hurriedly followed her words. Andrew never did ask why she was no longer sat opposite him, but he knew.

For Andrew's transplant to go ahead the hospital needed a suitable donor but, thus far, none had been found. They'd have daily discussions with the medical team at the hospital led by the amiable and comforting, Dr Joseph Humble. Always circulating, the veteran physician radiated an air of leadership in the department, Liz recognised his special attention to her and Andrew. Another doctor on the Gomer Berry Ward, by the name of 'Hobbs', was making noises about a possible donor from abroad, maybe Holland or

Belgium. It seemed a little risky, from Liz's perspective, and she'd been warned that it was a longshot, but she was open to all possibilities by this stage. The family took the decision to return home and wait in their own surroundings.

The next weeks saw Andrew in various states. His sandpit sat cold and undisturbed in the garden, he'd lost all interest in feeding the ducks or collecting buttercups at the park. His expression of resignation caused deep pain for anyone observing him. Yet, within days, he could be beside himself with boisterous laughter, making mud pies with his little brother, picking daisies or running down the path behind the house chasing an escaped goose.

After one of those good days of play in the garden he ran a fever and began complaining again of stomach pain. Soon enough, he was back in the confines of the stuffy cubicle, cared for by the nursing staff that had come to know him over the last year, at the children's hospital in London. The old record player made the journey to the hospital each time playing songs he never tired of: 'Three Blind Mice', 'Hickory Dickory Dock', 'Jack and Jill', and all his other favourites, over and over.

His pain was intense. He was vomiting blood, his veins regularly collapsed due to the demands of blood extraction, he was fed intravenously. Liz prayed for his death. The graphic horror had reached a stage that no parent ever wishes for, where death for your child is their source of least pain.

It was soon to be over. Liz and Roger kissed him goodnight as he slept on Friday 18th August and retreated upstairs, crossing paths with the ever-present Dr Humble, as they climbed to the green Mother's Unit on the top floor, with bedrooms available to parents of children being treated in the hospital. No sooner had they settled, a nurse scurried and rattled on the door, urging them to quickly return to the ward. When they arrived minutes later, Andrew was dead.

Liz held him in her arms. All signs of suffering were gone; his curls of burnished gold rested on his face and there was a feeling of indescribable peace. As she placed him back in the cot the realisation hit her like an unbelievable weight; an anchor plummeted through her body to the depths; initiating from the jaw, destructively thudding down indiscriminately through flesh, organs and bone until it sunk her to her knees. She wailed without tears. Her heart dismantled.

As the couple left the room sometime later, Liz noticed a nurse stood respectfully with tear-filled eyes in the corner. She'd been with Andrew until his last breath, comforting him as his life came to an end. Liz approached to offer whatever gratitude she could muster and asked if he'd said anything. "Another record", the nurse replied.

Caring for sick children
1972

"For goodness sake, we have to work as a team."
Ken Hugh-Jones' gaze remained low as half a dozen or so colleagues thundered passed him to leave the Tuesday morning meeting. Friction had been building for some time and was now forcing staff to take sides. Hugh-Jones' words, constituting the closing remarks and left unanswered, were a final plea, the culmination of a fraught few months at the Westminster Children's Hospital.

Silence blunted the scene. Wearily, Ken walked to the window and looked out over Vincent Square, at least able to savour the glow of morning sun. A hand rested on his shoulder; the chief mastermind of the latest fight trying to win favour. 'Such a piece of work', Ken muttered to himself. He was referring, as always, to Jack Hobbs.

Walking through the ward to begin his round of patient check-ins the usually enthusiastic consultant was forced to fake a smile. Children waved wearily at their passing doctor from plastic cocoons and wooden cubicles as parents devised new ways to keep them entertained. Ken, himself, had become weary. The internal combustion within his department was not only causing divisions, but personality clashes threatened to cause the whole unit to fall apart.

And the children around him were dying. A lot of them. Infants disappearing from existence unremarkably; at a rate painfully normalised. They were snowflakes landing in the ocean. His ward was full to capacity – around 108 beds - with young lives on the brink of death, every day each family facing unrivalled despair.

For the staff, the situation was a constant trial. Just a few years before, the Government had recorded statistics related to childhood blood cancer and disease, a primary cause of admission to Westminster Children's Hospital. Survival rate was calculated at around 5%. On average one child in every 10 diagnosed with a blood affected disease had a chance of survival into adulthood, the rest were highly likely to die. Blood cancer more generally accounted for one-third of all childhood cancers in Great Britain.

Consultant paediatrician, Dr Ken Hugh-Jones, had seen enough infant mortality to last him a lifetime and progress was proving too slow. Something was desperately needed to expedite a transformation. This was an immature field, seemingly in more ways than one. The NHS refused to invest in research of bone marrow transplantation given its substandard results thus, and pressure was on to hurry up or be forced to close down. Hugh-Jones and colleagues were forced to find other ways to fund this area of trial and error. And there was a lot of error; Ken's care of the children in the hospital was largely palliative. Without advancements in genuine treatment, it was about making children comfortable and supporting the families to find peace.

This wasn't the paediatrics Ken could stomach. Regardless of cost, and their own self-doubt, transplantation surely offered the only feasible way out of this mess. Within the bone marrow transplantation department, the team he'd assembled were capable and ambitious. You need an assortment of specialities to treat patients with these diseases, each as vital as the next for overall treatment outcomes, but immaturity saw them constantly at each other's throats. Each thinking their own approach superior, each aspiring for greatness, each disagreeing with the other's method. A typical personality clash: a combustible blend of ego, passion and ambition, surrounded entirely by infant mortality.

He needed to pull the battling factions together to meet on the same page. Success relied on partnership; without each other, they'd fail miserably, but they all believe their specialism to be the most important, their expertise to be more valuable. Failing a resolution, he needed to direct their conflict positively, to extract the best out of each another.

After storming out of the staff meeting ten-minutes earlier, Dr John Barrett buttoned up his woollen trench coat as he descended the main entrance steps onto Udall Street, took a left into the square and made his way towards the River Thames. He needed to clear his head. John wore his dark hair in a side parting, formal and fashionable; a charming young man enjoying professional and personal popularity in equal measure. London-life suited John. He relished meeting new people, approaching all liaisons with the confidence and assured demeanour afforded to a good-looking clinician in the city. Each passing day, however, increased his frustration. The fresh-faced haematologist was fairly new to the department, eager to make his name and John held an absolute conviction that his expertise was not only desirable for keeping these kids alive, but imperative.

Medicine hadn't always been on the cards. In fact, John hadn't shown any interest toward that career during school; enjoying sciences a normal amount but without the inclination that this may be his 'calling'. His mother, however, had always known. Her brother, Austin, was a brave medic that died in the war; his plane crashed and, despite surviving impact, an infection took hold and cost him his life. Retelling the story had always sparked young John's attention and, believing it to be the part about medicine rather than fighter pilots and the RAF, his mother was convinced he'd go on to treat the sick.

He attended St Bartholomew's Teaching Hospital, known as 'Barts', in London but felt quite out of place; all the students seemed to know each other, son or nephew of surgeons or consultants or whatever. John, the first of his family learning medicine, felt somewhat of a country bumkin. He was getting by just fine though, achieving his grades and sleepwalking himself towards a career of some description.

That is until he spent a semester in South Africa. It was the late 1960s; the Border War with Namibia, Angola and Zambia had begun; children, in their hundreds, were dying in front of his eyes of totally curable diseases. They'd arrive at the clinic with measles, malaria, malnourishment and diarrhoea and, within days, he'd be consoling their parents. Or, conversely on occasion, play a crucial role seeing them on the road to recovery.

This is the moment John stopped *playing* at medicine. He realised that he was needed.

Immersed in the life and death of blood, John Barrett merged the study of haematology with a newfound passion for saving children. Nowhere was this calling more pertinent than at the Westminster Children's Hospital.

Treating sick children: a new concept

A belief that medical care concerning children should use distinctly different methods from those of treating adults dates back as far back as Hippocrates, the 'Father of Medicine', in 400 BC. It's thought he was first to reference the unique physiology of the infant and the distinct nutritional and medical needs of the growing child. Paediatrics, the area of medicine focused on caring for children, infants and adolescents, can actually be traced back to texts in Ancient India. Then came Persian philosopher and physician Abū Bakr Muhammad ibn Zakariyyā al-Rāzī (865–925 AD), an early polymath who published an essay on paediatrics titled 'Diseases in Children' as well as offering the first definite description of smallpox as a clinical entity. The first time paediatrics was written about as a medical specialism was by Swedish physician Nils Rosén von Rosenstein in 1764. Following a period as the King of Sweden's chief physician, he wrote *The Diseases of Children, and their Remedies* – considered to be the first textbook on the subject.

It was to be a further 40-years until the Western world's first hospital dedicated solely to the treatment of children was created in a European city where, at the time, half of *all* children died before the age of 10.

Suzanne Necker (nee Curchod), a Swiss-born salonist, founded the Hospice de Charité in Paris in 1778 in a move to reform overcrowded hospitals by building smaller treatment centres closer to where people lived. Hospitals at the time were dismal. French Encyclopaedist Denis Diderot described Hôtel-Dieu de Paris, the city's oldest, as: "the biggest, roomiest, richest and most terrifying of all hospitals. Imagine every kind of patient, sometimes packed three, four, five, or six into a bed, living alongside the dead and dying, the air polluted by this mass of sick bodies, passing the pestilential germs of their affections from one to the other, and the spectacle of suffering and agony on every hand." While perhaps offering better conditions the new charity hospital, located in a disused monastery, was run by Nuns rather than doctors and surgeons; their menu more palliative than scientific. To even get through the doors you needed to show your baptism certificate and practice confession. But alongside her husband, Jacques Necker, who worked as head of the French finance ministry under King Louis XVI, they developed this 'hospital' where patients of all ages, regardless of wealth, could go to be treated, or to comfortably die. 'Madame Necker', as she was known, spoke of her very clear aims: "to show the possibility of nursing sick people, each one in a bed to himself, with all the care dictated by the kindliest humanity, without exceeding a fixed price."

This was not, however, a great time to be closely aligned with the King.

In 1789, Louis XVI took interventionist steps to subdue a rebellious group that felt themselves oppressed by the aristocracy and monarchy. He closed down their usual meeting place and, as a result, these rebels met on a tennis court in Versailles to devise a plan that would amount to the French Revolution. A few weeks after the 'Tennis Court Oath', the King dismissed his popular minister, Necker, and, just two days later, a crowd of armed Parisians stormed the Bastille and the revolution began.

Years of bloody battle ripped through France with the abolition of the monarchy, formation of a republic and political turmoil until the end of the century.

Which is why Paris in 1801 seems a curious time to introduce the world's first ever hospital exclusively for the treatment of sick children.

The Hôpital des Enfants-Malades was established on the Rue de Sévres, adjoining Madame Necker's now renamed Hospice de l'Ouest, with a clear remit to care "for the children of both sexes under the age of fifteen years". Previously a work shelter for around 100 poor women, then used for coal storage during the Revolution, and subsequently as an orphanage for Parisian children. A decree came down to relocate the children of the Maison Nationale des

Orphelins to elsewhere in the city and to prepare the building to become the first hospital of its kind in history.

Over the next 50-years the hospital had great successes developing the study of paediatric diseases, development, and nutrition and, by 1850, had grown to have 600 beds to treat sick children. In the mid-1830s, a student of medicine visiting from England spent time working at the Parisian children's hospital gathering a deeper understanding of why treating children and infants in a more specialised way had such benefit. On his return to London, Dr Charles West, another graduate of St Bartholomew's Hospital like John Barrett, set about persuading the London medical establishment that setting up a hospital specifically for children and infants had medical merit. Throughout the 1840s, alongside his physician post at the Waterloo Road Dispensary for Women and Children[12], West pleaded to every person with sway in physician circles to support his passion. He desperately wanted an inpatient hospital dedicated to the care of sick children. By 1850, after a decade of relentless lobbying and countless setbacks, powerful people began to listen.

In the face of much derision from peers, the Spring of 1851 saw Dr West open the doors to Great Britain's first children's hospital, at number 49 Great Ormond Street.

Great Ormond Street Hospital – Britain's first hospital for sick children

The first child treated was three-year old Eliza Armstrong, in

---

[12] A dispensary was a type of hospital that was able to administer drugs. In this instance the hospital was like a modern-day maternity unit

February 1852. Her parents had made the journey across town pushing her by pram all the way from Little James Street – literally a few minutes' walk from the front gates of Buckingham Palace, recently refurbished and inhabited by its first monarch, Queen Victoria. Records show that Eliza stayed at hospital for five-days as an out-patient suffering from Phthisis, an old term for what is now known as Tuberculosis; a diagnosis that makes it highly unlikely Eliza would have survived.

West's Hospital for Sick Children started out with just ten beds but as word got out, and parents brought their children to be treated, his numbers tripled from 1,252 out-patient treatments in the first year, to 4,251 the next and again rising to around perhaps 8,000 in year-three. It was quite hands on in those early days, for everyone; the first patients' families were allowed to help with their children's treatment, with only five nurses to cover day and night shifts. Medical knowledge at the time meant little could be done to cure young patients. For many, however desperate this may sound, a stay at the hospital will have provided them a wash, substantial food and warmth; something their poverty in the Victorian era will almost certainly not have otherwise allowed. If being in a hospital bed made a difference at all, it was those comforts plus attentive, friendly care. Whether you survived or not depended on the natural history of the disease itself. 'Medicine' made little or no difference.

Despite having managed to increase the number of in-patient beds to 30, West was focused on securing further funds to support more of London's sick, and poor, children. He also had a keen eye for politics and health inequalities, if this quote is anything to go by: "Thirty beds! when more than 21,000 children die every year in this metropolis under ten years of age; and when this mortality falls thrice as heavily on the poor as on the rich! But alas, the tables of mortality do not tell the whole of the sad tale. It is not only because so many children die, that this Hospital was founded; but because so many are sick; because they languish in their homes; a burden to their parents who have no leisure to tend them, no means to minister to their wants. The one sick child weighs down the whole family; it keeps the father poor, the home wretched."

The Hospital navigated its first financial crisis in 1858 with the help of a friend of Dr West, Charles Dickens; he was navigating his own personal crisis at the time, separating from his wife to be with 18-year-old actress, Ellen Ternan. Dickens threw himself into the project, perhaps as a distraction, with a series of public readings at St. Martin-in-the-Fields church hall which landed the hospital back on a solid footing. One evening alone, 9th February 1858, Dickens' readings brought in around £3,000 in donations (something in the region of £420,000 today). With the money, the hospital purchased the neighbouring house, 48 Great Ormond Street, increasing the bed capacity from 30 to 75.

By the 1870s, Dr Charles West had stepped back from activity at the hospital but the foundations he laid would eventually prove pivotal in treating child illness in London. Yet even by the end of the century, the ability to cure sick children remained largely unattainable. On 18th April 1895, a 17-month-old boy called Percy was admitted to the Hospital for Sick Children and given a diagnosis, according to his medical notes, of *leucocythaemia* – an early description of leukaemia. Like many thousands of children turning up to the hospital in the decades before and after him this diagnosis offered zero chance of survival and, within 12-days, little Percy was dead. *Leucocythaemia* was proving to be the biggest killer of children entering the hospital, aside from accidents, and while surgeons tried to tackle some other forms of cancer by cutting the solid tumours out, leukaemia was simply decided to be incurable.

British children are dying

In 1903, another children's hospital opened its doors in London; the St Francis Hospital for Infants, later renamed The Infants Hospital, at 7 Denning Road, right next to the beautiful open fields of Hampstead Heath. It assumed control of a building already caring for children and was founded by physician Dr Ralph Vincent and the local Mond family to care for children and infants in the Camden area. At the time there had been little improvement in infant mortality rates since Great Ormond Street opened over 50-years earlier. In fact, Dr Vincent claimed that 24% of the total deaths in England and Wales in the year 1900 were infants under the age of one year. That's a quarter of *all* deaths – not just infant deaths.

Helena Edith Levis, or Edith as she preferred to be known, had met her husband-to-be, Sir Robert Ludwig Mond, when she was volunteering as a secretary at this very clinic in Hampstead in 1897. She was desperate to understand how they could reduce infant mortality and, when he visited the project as a funder that year, the pair were introduced. Many of the deaths were linked to infant malnutrition and again we see leading thinkers making attributions to class divides, with George Carpenter, founder of the British Journal of Children's Diseases, claiming that infant mortality "does not exist to any serious extent in the upper and middle class".

So, an institution "dedicated to the care of babies from working-class families in their first weeks and months appeared absolutely essential to address the problem"[xiv]. Edith and Dr Vincent led a committee of wealthy men and women with the objective of setting up such an institution. It was a strong partnership: Dr Ralph Vincent was meticulous in his research into infant nutrition through cow's milk and other alternatives; while Edith, with the financial and social backing to make their vision a reality, recruited benefactors to support their cause. They both worked tirelessly, day and night, to provide a fighting chance for these children.

When the doors opened in 1903 a newspaper wrote: "The Hospital was founded for scientific treatment of young babies suffering from malnutrition, and it was the aim of the committee to make it a centre for treatment of infantile diseases, for the study of all factors connected with the rearing of a strong people[xv]."

Edith devoted herself to caring for the young patients, making an environment that gave them a fighting chance at life. But two years later tragedy entered the home. The relentless emotional strain of caring for deeply sick children became increasingly difficult to bear for Edith. Her sleep had become interrupted, her mind constantly raced. She wasn't a mother herself but felt maternal responsibility for each and every child patient. When she did doze off, she was blighted by terrors of screaming babies, their eyes wide, turning to her for salvation. The noises of the hospital ward would ring in her ears, she could find no release, and her doctor prescribed pills to help induce sleep. Over the Christmas period, in 1905, Edith joined her husband on an archaeological exploration trip to Egypt. She desperately needed the break. On 28th December she took her sleeping tablets, desperate for a morsel of peace, an escape from the torment, just for an instant. She overdosed. Edith, just 32 years old, was found dead the next morning. She died alone, her final moments in isolation, something she'd worked so hard to avoid for the children[xvi].

Devastated by his wife's passing, Robert Mond decided to build in a brand-new children's hospital in her name, as a memorial to Edith's unrelenting commitment to infants in London. With investment from members of the Mond family and private sponsors (around 75% being women), they constructed a new Infants

Hospital in Vincent Square, Westminster, in 1907.

Death square

Having walked along the riverbank towards the Houses of Parliament, John Barrett re-entered Vincent Square from the north, passing the Royal Oak pub via Horseferry Road. It always bothered him knowing that the people inside the Palace of Westminster could save more children's lives with the stroke of a pen at the foot of a cheque than he could through his own graft on the front line. Just the way it was intended, his pragmatism decided. As the crow flies, from his entry point to the hospital directly in front of him across the square, would take no time at all to walk. But black iron railings encasing the central grass area required circumnavigating; used for cricket, football and tennis by the local school. On days like today, as autumnal sun pierced gaps between buildings, glowing lines toning the grass and intermittent warmth reaching his cheeks, he didn't mind the extra walk.

The resplendent central field of Vincent Square, just outside the Westminster Children's Hospital, wasn't always used for school sports. Back in time the area was known as Tothill Fields, but the reason for the name is up for debate. Some believe it originates from 'Teut', the place 'where solemn proclamations were made to the people'[13] and, being an elevated part of the area, 'Tut-hill' was often heard as 'Tuttle'. The Normans, however, spoke of these parts as "Thorny Island, et tout la champ", meaning 'and all the field'. If you lazily Anglicise these latter words, you may be left with something sounding like 'Tuttle'.

---

[13] https://www.british-history.ac.uk/old-new-london/vol4/pp14-26

This location is the epicentre of this story. Buried below the seemingly quintessential English square, with pristinely mowed lawns smelling lusciously fresh, are foundations of untold darkness and rot, the like of which we'd perhaps prefer to leave forgotten. But we're here now, so let's take a little look.

Digging up the grass roots, through perfectly cultivated strands, would reveal the rotten, discarded remains of an abandoned wasteland, burned out belongings and jagged metal relics. Purchased in exchange for a horse and plough by the Dean of Westminster, William Vincent, the Badlands were in a state of neglect in the 18th century, used at that time only by local children as a makeshift playground. Buried under another layer of earth, beneath the feet of these children as they played, notorious convicted criminals traipsed the dark corridors of Tothill Fields Bridlewell prison, locked up and serving their time in conditions as dank and lowly as you can imagine.

Once a penitentiary, depriving liberty and embodying the brutality of the age, chain clangs and whip snaps echoed through the air. This marshy tract of land, lying between Millbank and Westminster Abbey, has yet more buried layers; one more exhumation would uncover the remains of battle-worn bears, thrown into the square's central ring to bite, to claw, to roar; blood-sport for the entertainment of Queen Anne of England and Ireland, and amusement of fellow onlookers.

Standing in the pen, bears raged helplessly as vicious dogs snapped at their heels. The soil beneath their paws was a deep purple, permeating the unmistakable stench of death. A tier deeper into the annals of history will reveal a horde of corpses; a teeming pit filled with bodies overlapping without order, all tortured victims of the Great Plague of London. The year they succumbed is 1665. It's difficult to ascertain the quota; quite how many souls the angularly strewn body parts can be attributed to. We're passing them by, their moment of recognition brief as we focus on those that came before them; barely cold.

Welcome to the death camp.

Prisoners captured in the Battle of Worcester 1651, where Oliver Cromwell's army defeated Charles II's Royalists, were either deported or locked up. Most were Scottish, shackled here in the square far from home, starved to death and buried where they fell. The depths of our knowledge about Vincent Square lie just one further level down, in the Middle Ages, where it's much more sparse and very little exists around but a scattering of shacks among wide open fields through to the river and beyond. On a mound of earth raised in the square, a necromancer stands trial. The charge is witchcraft; conjuring spirits of the dead brought fear among the living that they were being used as some sort of weapon. Summoned spirits would watch on as the trial concluded, scattered before them instruments of the trade, banished and destroyed, bringing an end to the death magic they invoke.

John, unknowing, left the chaotic history behind, rounding the corner back onto Udall Street; buried mortality now filled in behind him, the ever-present fate of his work loomed in his eyeline, ascending the steps at the main entrance of the Westminster Children's Hospital.

How do you fight an invisible killer?

Swapping out his coats, lab replacing woollen, John pulled his stool into position. He'd hardly eaten anything all day, rarely did if he was pushed, but was far too worked up for lunch. He moved his microscope close, took his selection of cells in culture from the incubator and slid them into acute view.

As a leading haematologist in the department, Barrett fixed his attention on understanding the mesmeric nuances of the circulatory system. The beauty of blood had become his obsession. At any given moment, each person has 1.2 gallons of blood (around 10% of your total body weight) gallantly traversing the body delivering oxygen to cells and taking away carbon dioxide in exchange. On its rounds it drops off crucial nutrients, including vitamins, glucose, amino acids and minerals while also playing an important role in moderating our body temperature, expanding or contracting blood vessels to move blood closer or farther from the skin surface (where temperature cools).

Blood is a fluid tissue, not simply fluid, due to the amount of living cells active in the circulating plasma. Within this fluid tissue also exists platelets; not full cells but fragments of cells that kick into action when we cut ourselves, rapidly clumping around the damaged area to form a plug, or clot, to stop the blood escaping the body.

All this aside, when John squints through the optic in the lab his attention is always on the white blood cells, also known as leukocytes. Their job is to fight all infections, yet they make up only 1% of all blood circulating our body. Despite their low numbers they're pretty good at it. When these white blood cells start to go wrong, however, the whole intricate operation begins to fall apart.

Children at the Westminster Children's Hospital were admitted for a wide variety of sickness and disease but one third of all admissions were specifically blood disease related. They'd first pioneered bone marrow transplantation (BMT) back in the 1950s, using cells obtained from the same patient, to try saving them from faulty immune systems. Almost always, it failed. Blood disease, in all its many varieties, was proving tricky to get to grips with.

Haematologists focus on many variations of immunodeficiencies but also on three main types of blood cancer: lymphoma, myeloma and leukaemia. All forms occur when the white blood cells begin to falter, effectively leaving your body a bit of an open target for disease to strike.

Lymphoma is defined as either Hodgkin's or non-Hodgkin's: mostly affecting adults, and predominantly those aged over 40. The name comes from Thomas Hodgkin, a pathologist who, in 1832, wrote an understated report that went largely unnoticed for many years about his observations of seven patients with enlarged lymph nodes. Hodgkin's lymphoma is considered more treatable as it hinges on the presence of an abnormal cell, which can be spotted under the microscope and targeted. Non-Hodgkin's lymphoma could arise in any lymph nodes in the body and is often diagnosed at a more advanced stage making it less treatable.

Myeloma occurs in the plasma cells in our blood; these cells produce antibodies in the form of proteins so, when we get sick through an infection, plasma cells begin producing antibodies, dependent on which infection we have, to attack and kill the bacteria or virus. When things go wrong in myeloma cells they produce an irregular form of one type of antibody, impotent and powerless to strike infections. There are many names for these antibodies including abnormal proteins, paraproteins, monoclonal proteins, or a monoclonal spike. These ineffective cells crop up in numerous areas at once where bone marrow is active, often seeing it referred to as multiple myeloma.

Leukaemia is the most common type of blood cancer, especially when the patient is a child. It forms in the lymphocyte cells in the bone marrow, the factory where all blood cells originate, and sees faulty white blood cells created in out-of-control numbers. Not only are these cells unable to properly do their job but in such large numbers they flood the space, stifling the bone marrow's ability to produce red blood cells which keep our organs working effectively.

There are a few types of leukaemia, one of the most common found in children being *Acute Lymphoblastic Leukaemia* (referred to as 'ALL').

Given we're talking a lot here about the complexities of blood – something people study for years (and realistically their whole careers) to fully understand – it's worth breaking down some of the functionalities in terms perhaps a little less science-heavy.

So, the white blood in our system, or lymphocyte cells, come in two forms. The first of which is a B cell: the security guard or bouncer on the door of the local nightclub. When they see an altercation beginning at the entrance to their establishment they spring into action, producing a protein called an antibody which latches on and destroys any invading viruses or bacteria before they get chance to infect other cells. The other type is a T cell: these are the kamikaze fighters, unafraid to see a bit of collateral damage. They spot when an invasion has taken place, perhaps the cunning virus evaded the bouncers and slipped passed the B-cells, causing a bit of a ruckus and taking control of some of the body's own cells. At this point the walkie talkies go off and the T cells step in, proceeding to destroy the culprits plus any of the body's indigenous cells that have become infected.

It's an effective system and keeps our body infection free. A problem arises when these B and T cells stop maturing at the normal rate and go into overdrive, proliferating at a much quicker ratio. This creates a huge build-up of these malfunctioning white cells in the bone marrow.

John Barrett had a serious issue with these faulty cells. So effective when on song but ruinous if out of control. They were the reason so many children were dying before his eyes. He knew it, and the team knew it, but they didn't know how to stop it.

The cycle played out excruciatingly like clockwork. If you receive a heart or liver transplant, you can continue to live with someone else's organ inside you. If accepted by the body, this new piece of kit can happily acclimatise to its new surroundings and operate in perfect harmony. The same applies with blood. What pumps through your veins and arteries when the transplant is successful is someone else's blood, only it is now produced inside your body. The blood stem cells discovered by *Till and McCulloch*, those super cells capable of producing a wide array of others like themselves, are creating fresh replicas in their new blood factory. After a week, however, things start to go wrong. A child's skin starts to speckle and blister on the surface, red and sore, before flaking off at a touch. The child vomits without warning, stops eating and suffers green and watery diarrhoea. The infant's skin and the whites of the eyes begin to turn yellow with jaundice and, soon after, the child dies from multiple organ failure.

For John and the transplant team, this process was observed time and again. The young children didn't know what was happening to them; neither did the doctors or nurses, who'd transplanted what they believed to be a matched solution. They watched as these small lives shrank and disappeared before them. Say what you want about the bedside manner of doctors, or the flippancy of a Registrar, they felt the pain.

John was struggling to concentrate; frustration from the earlier meeting persisted. He stepped away from the microscope; time to visit the basement.

The team at Westminster Children's Hospital had started to devote a little more time into the intricacies of a new discovery, called HLA. Or, as the practice was more commonly known, tissue typing. John reached a broom cupboard in the basement and knocked twice on the green painted door. He was immediately summoned in.

Hounded from the inside, out

Tucked away, bothering no one, in his untroubled corner of the basement was Dr David James. Blood Transfusion Officer at the Westminster Hospital, Dr James cast a tall but unassuming figure. He wore thick-rimmed glasses, dark-brown hair combed over the few remaining whisps clinging to the top of his head, and he spoke softly but purposefully with a gentle Welsh-twang. He had a senior full-time role in the hospital ensuring all transplants had correct and sufficient blood supply. In his "spare time", however, he'd created a makeshift lab in a small broom cupboard below the hospital where, at any given opportunity, he would squirrel himself away to develop his understanding of this new area of science that no one really gave much resource to. And the lack of investment showed. Aside from the cupboard, which had space enough for one lab bench and basic borrowed equipment, there was an 'office' of sorts fashioned in an alcove under the stairwell. The records of donors were scribbled out, filed on small index cards and stored in a shoebox.

All this aside, Drs James and Barrett knew the importance of developing this line of haematological enquiry. They were desperate. What the children were dying from was Graft versus Host Disease (GvHD). OK, here's a term you're going to hear a few times in this story and its discovery is a crucial milestone in the history of blood disease.

Understanding this phenomenon was to be significantly important in transforming survival rates and one of the primary reasons blood was drastically more complex to graft. Graft versus Host pertains to the *graft*, in this case the new blood, rejecting the host body it now dwelled in.

Consider again a patient that receives a new heart. After a week or two of becoming acclimatised it sometimes occurs that the body simply rejects this alien organ as a trespasser. The T-cells in our immune system see the foreign object as a direct threat and decide they must destroy the intruder. They attack the heart cells until, if left for long enough, it is no longer fit for purpose. The organ rejected its back to the drawing board for the medical team who must find another replacement organ and hope this one has more success. In this instance, they can whip it out and try again; another organ may be greeted with a warmer reception.

When the transplant is blood stem cells, the rejection process is exactly the opposite.

The new blood, now produced inside the bones and circulating the body, is creating all the functioning cells the old faulty blood could not. A few weeks in and the new immune system has sent its operational white blood cells to all corners of the body. It doesn't take long to realise that their surroundings are somewhat unfamiliar. To the immune system the trespasser, in this instance, is the body itself, or the 'host'. Time for those kamikaze T-cells in the blood to do what they do best when a threat is spotted; they begin to attack. By now widespread in the person, they systematically strike against organs, starting with those connected to the outside world like the skin, liver, eyes and gut. A Trojan horse, of sorts, the stems cells are an unknown foe that have been welcomed into the inner sanctum, fortified gates closed behind them. Originally invited, but now very much unwanted guests, these white blood cells set about annihilating their host and putting the body under siege. Over the course of a few weeks the immune system takes total control, shutting down the core functions of its host body, meticulously and painfully killing the person from the inside-out. The invaders triumphant, it's game over.

A pretty grim realisation, especially when physicians had chosen to put this graft in the patient. But Dr David James had noticed something important. While many children were dying of Graft vs Host Disease, he'd observed that twins were not. When the graft was exchanged between almost identically matching genes the success rate was vastly improved. There was something in this. The closer matched these HLA antigens, or tissue type, of donor and recipient, the lower the likelihood of rejection? That perhaps the body couldn't as easily differentiate between self and non-self if the HLA was distractingly similar. Could they trick the body into accepting similar blood? If there were no identical siblings, how similar could you get away with?

It was a basement side hustle, not something his employer specifically paid him to research, but Dr James was eager to explore tissue typing further.

It needed testing. That required more samples for his shoebox. A lot more.

Leave your deposits at the bank
1972

"Our beloved angel left us at around 1am. He looked the most perfect, perfect person I have ever seen when I last saw him in this earthly world."

Pain unrivalled. Liz's diary entry on 18th August 1972 was brief and to-the-point. She no longer cried; instead, her body shook. She thought she'd have escaped the horrid, sterile confines of the hospital at the first opportunity but found herself unable to walk out through the door. She felt Andrew was still there, close-by. She couldn't leave him.

When her dad Denis arrived the next morning to take Liz and Roger home in his car, his eyes were red, sore and bloodshot. She'd never known him to cry before. Stepping through their front door at Welham Green, Liz was deafened by the silence. Andrew would never be here again. A friend had taken Simon out for a walk, a distraction, but Mollie was waiting, arms outstretched.

"I'm alright. I really am perfectly alright." Liz knew hugging her mother would open the floodgates. She began to brainwash herself. Tell herself that grieving would make others unhappy and that was the last thing Andrew would have wanted. Such a happy child deserves a happy mother.

The first few days were the worst. She remembered how beautiful he was when dead. How his shape and weight felt in her arms. The suffering had left him alone, finally. She tried to find thanks for that. "Please God, make life easier for us to bear', she diarised soon after. 'I feel, although I grieve, that my one is safe with you somewhere." The funeral was small, at Golders Green Crematorium in north London. As always, she confided in her diary, "we said farewell to our precious baby at 1:45pm today. It was a beautiful service."

Her fierce and protective style of love now focused only upon Simon. Liz decided against returning to her job. With her second boy increasingly sick, and her husband undergoing difficult treatment himself, she compartmentalised grief and fixated on being productive. She'd consume repetitive tasks within the house; cooking, cleaning, bills, gardening, cleaning, cooking, minor renovations, cleaning. All the while watching, bathing, feeding, medicating and playing with her little boy. It kept her mind focused on things she *could* control.

Seclusion gave her opportunity to think about having another child, the doctors had even suggested it. Far from being a replacement, they'd explained, if it were a girl, she would certainly not inherit the same disease. She'd be a healthy baby. And if a boy, well, they'd have the option to terminate. When Liz posed the question to Roger, more bad news. He revealed the drugs he was taking to treat his cancer had made him sterile; he'd found out on the day of Andrew's funeral but had told no one.

Loneliness wasn't exclusive to daylight hours. She was sleeping very little; thinking incessantly, all night through, and the darkest hours revealed the darkest thoughts in her mind. Maybe she'd accuse herself of murder; actively bringing children into the world only for them to die by her genetic defects. Roger was to blame too. Perhaps he hated the devotion she had for their boys, he felt rejected. That is why he got cancer; to compete for her affection.

Those thoughts were irrational by morning but intensely real at night. The resulting tiredness made her snappy. She started drinking in the evenings, just a little nightcap once Simon had gone to bed. A Vermouth helped to take the edge off, settle her thoughts. It barely changed the outcome. The peaks and troughs of mood magnified. Some days Mollie would turn up after Roger went to work and found Simon, in his pyjamas, playing alone quite contently on his bedroom floor. She'd find Liz bound to her bed, filled with worry, nerves and weakening low mood.

It resurfaced the debilitating depression she experienced as a teen, that led her to residential stays at an institution. Liz reached out to medics for support, this time for herself.

Her GP prescribed a new drug called Diazepam, a form of antidepressant, to ease the imbalance. They had only recently been introduced to the market, freely distributed on the NHS, and were being dished out like sweets. They worked well for Liz, taking away her brain power and allowing her mind to rest and recuperate. Alongside the Vermouth, evenings became sedate. Those close to her worried but felt they needed to cut her some slack. Whichever method she chose to cope with this hellish situation was OK with them.

From one unthinkable trial to the immediate next.

Simon's body grumbled under the pressure of his faulty blood. He was weak, often erupting in irritating rashes and painful ulcers with seeming nonchalance. Living with an immune deficiency, Simon's blood was lacking something to protect him. His infection fighting cells, the soldiers of the blood known as neutrophils, lacked the ammo to effectively kill enemy bacteria or fungal infections. They had the guns, but they fired blanks. For children diagnosed with blood cancer, like leukaemia, they needed something a little more.

Their immunity cells were present but dangerous; they needed switching off and replacing to give any chance of survival. A somewhat different challenge needing somewhat different treatment.

What the Bostic family now knew, to avoid what happened to Andrew, was that Simon's survival depended on a stranger. That one person in 50,000 needed to come forward and be willing to donate their stem cells in an effort to save his life.

*

It's one thing to donate your blood or an organ to a close family member. If your own child, or a relative, desperately needed your help to live it may be the easiest decision in the world to donate. Would people, however, decide to offer that same bodily donation to a person they had never met and may never meet.

In the 1970s, as the Bostic family navigated this new stem cell world, the concept of voluntary blood and organ donation was relatively new.

'Blood banks', a term coined by Dr Bernard Fantus, were first set up across the UK and USA in 1937. Fantus, director of therapeutics at the Cook County Hospital in Chicago, established America's first blood bank at his hospital and more popped up across the country throughout the year. The notion had been made possible a few years earlier, in 1932, when Russian physician, Dr Andre Bagdasarov, managed to store blood for an incredible 21-days. Prior to this, efforts to keep blood 'alive' and on stand-by had all failed miserably but Bagdasarov kept it strictly at four-degrees centigrade, adding a measured quantity of glucose with sodium citrate, thus creating the world's first blood bank.

Timing of the discovery was opportune.

When World War II broke out, in 1939, there was a new and

enormous need for transfusions. Blood donation centres sprang up across Britain asking the public to do their bit for the war effort and donate blood for soldiers on the frontline. Transfusions themselves were another recent discovery. It was only at the beginning of the Spanish Civil War, in 1936, that doctor, Federic Durán-Jordà, established the world's first transfusion service in Barcelona. For the 'greater good', people in Britain turned up and queued at their nearest blood bank, had a needle inserted into their arm and deposited around 2/3 pint of their blood. Donors, normal civilians who sometimes felt they were helpless in the fight, would leave knowing their blood would be sent to surgeons on the battlefields, having a direct impact on the war.

To that end, pioneer Charles R. Drew developed the "Plasma for Britain" program — a pilot project in the United States collecting blood for shipment to their allies across the Atlantic. Awarded a Rockefeller Fellowship in surgery in 1938 at Columbia University, Drew researched at Columbia's Presbyterian Hospital and wrote a doctoral thesis entitled, "Banked Blood: A Study on Blood Preservation[xvii]". Excitingly, his research found that by separating plasma (the liquid part of blood) from the whole blood (where all the other cells, including red and white blood cells, exist) and then refrigerating them separately, blood lasted longer and was less likely to become contaminated[xviii]. In the five-month project, Drew set the standard for clean transfusions of plasma overseeing donations from 5,000 people and sending over 5,500 vials of blood plasma to Britain.

Within all the newly donated litres of blood slushing around, plasma was the prime ingredient.

It was believed that as the body goes into shock both blood pressure and body temperature decrease causing a lack of blood flow and a loss of oxygen in the body's tissues and cells. Transfusing plasma staved off shock and bleeding, allowing time for the soldier to reach medical care.

Journalist Ernie Pyle spent time on the frontline in World War II and was repeatedly asked by surgeons to tell people back home about the wonders of plasma. They deemed it "absolutely magical" and "the outstanding medical discovery of the war"[xix].[14]

Blood transfusions were now seen to be a key ingredient for public health, not just in war but for operations taking place at home. But many more blood donations were needed. In 1946, the Ministry of Health took control of Britain's blood banks, setting up the National Blood Transfusion Service[xx] and, just two-years later, the National Health Service (NHS) was founded, offering universal health care, free at the point of delivery. A public information film in 1949 explained how this important new 'savings bank' stored something much more vital than money, with "life-giving blood and plasma". It even used the story of young boy, Raymond Charles - a precursor to future media campaigns – whose life had been saved due to a blood transfusion from the donations register[xxi].

When soldiers were in need, people chose to line the street at blood banks to give away something very personal and sacred to

---

[14] Ernest Pyle wrote articles and broadcast a radio show, 'Life to the Front', to raise public awareness of the important impact their donation could have in the war effort. Until this point the immediate benefits of plasma transfusion hadn't been fully known but, in practice, were proving to save lives.

potentially save the life of a stranger.[15] But what does it take to donate organs or blood? Do donors seek the warm glow that comes from a socially positive act, or was it just reluctant altruism; the knowledge that many others were doing the same and they didn't wish to be an outlier?

As Liz squared up to the challenge in 1972, she knew that encouraging people into voluntary donation was something modern medicine, and civil society, was consistently working on. For strangers to give their precious blood. If this was the child of another mother, what would inspire Liz to donate? She'd need to hear their story; the heartache, the injustice, the necessary steps to rescue. Then she could invest, both her emotions and her blood.

---

[15] Since 1616, when Dr William Harvey demonstrated systemic circulation of blood around the brain and body by the heart, scientists have grappled with how to cure the ills caused by blood. In 1665, Dr Richard Lower performed the first animal to animal blood transfusion between two dogs but, when he and others subsequently trialled animal to human transfusions, there were several unnecessary deaths.

Supress your instincts
1960

Dr Hardisty had seen dead bodies before. His father had died very young, he'd completed National Service abroad at the end of the war and, as part of his training, had spent more time than he'd originally anticipated with dying patients on the wards of St Thomas' Teaching Hospital in London.

He'd seen plenty of dead bodies, but there was something particularly daunting about what he saw in his new job. Tiny bodies expiring from this microscopically visible, yet untouchable, cancer. This was the harsh reality facing the 36-year-old doctor, newly charged as the first consultant haematologist at the Hospital for Sick Children, Great Ormond Street.

Since 17-month-old Percy died in the very same building, over 60 years before, very little had changed for those diagnosed with childhood leukaemia. Clean-shaven and wearing distinctive thick half-rimmed glasses, Roger Hardisty (not to be confused with Simon's father, Roger Bostic) walked through the doors to his new job in 1958 as an expert in investigating diseases in blood. He actually had no formal training in paediatrics but the success of the unit was his responsibility. A quiet and modest man, Hardisty was a dreamer; he strongly believed a cure for childhood leukaemia was possible but, as things stood, the death rate for those diagnosed was 100%. And he didn't quite know where to begin.

"It's like climbing Everest with little equipment or knowledge of how to get to the top", someone mused to Hardisty when he explained that he planned to tackle leukaemia.

"But you never know if you'll achieve it if you don't set off", he'd reply.

A northern girl named, Susan

Six-weeks after Susan Eastwood was diagnosed with leukaemia, in 1960, she was dead.

Described by family as a 'giggly' Teesside girl, Susan relentlessly pursued fun. She'd plead that her older sister push her higher and higher on their back garden swing, would play for hours with family dog, Whiskey, and run along the nearby beaches at every opportunity. Neighbours in her family's community of Middlesbrough were well-aware of her vivacity so when news circulated of this little-known illness it came as quite a shock. Over the weeks her energy levels sapped. Drugs caused her face to swell and puff, her skin colour and spirits equally drained, and fatigue weakened her with each passing day. "I think I will have a little sleep on my bed", she'd tell her mother, Hilda, not so long after finishing breakfast.

Just a few weeks shy of her seventh birthday, Susan's short life was over. A diagnosis of acute lymphoblastic leukaemia (ALL) in 1960s Teesside was a death sentence. Even if they'd had found their way down to Dr Roger Hardisty's office at Great Ormond Street in London, the leading centre for childhood disease, Susan's chances would likely have been the same. After all, even *their* survival rate for childhood leukaemia at the time was 0%.

As Susan departed this world, the Eastwood family remained behind, wrestling grief; an uninvited guest that now engulfed their lives. While courting the searing pain of losing a child, they privately mused incredulity that this cancer was untouchable. Those fighting other forms of cancer were achieving better results every year. How could it be that so little was understood about treatment for cancer of the blood?

In their small front room in the weeks following Susan's death, mother Hilda and sister Sylvia started sewing pocket handkerchiefs to pieces of card that slid neatly inside the breast pocket of a suit jacket. The new fashion trend was a distraction. Father David organised whip arounds at work and the family produced Christmas cards with proceeds going to charity, something that was quite unheard of beforehand. There was no clear plan but Susan's parents wanted their daughter's short life to have some greater meaning. Selling pocket hankies locally could raise a bit of money and perhaps help experts find out more about this mysterious illness.

Pretty soon donations started to pour in. Hilda and David formalised their fundraising appeal by setting up a charity with a goal of researching this fatal disease. If they could contribute, even in a small way to finding a cure, then Susan's death would have had deeper meaning. In their daughter's name they set up the 'Leukaemia Research Fund' in Teesside.

Local and national media quickly picked up the story and the appeal took on a life of its own. No longer focused on handkerchiefs, donations from the public had raised £3,000 (about £50,000 in today's money) within a year and it was time to decide how best to invest it. The Eastwoods read an article in 'The People' magazine highlighting the importance of research into childhood diseases at The Hospital for Sick Children and, with that, the decision was made. A few letters and phone calls later and an agreement was in place. They would fund the creation of the first ever dedicated ward to search for a cure for leukaemia.

On a Saturday morning in December 1961, Dr Roger Hardisty welcomed the Eastwoods to his new ward at Great Ormond Street for the official unveiling. Their incredible and unexpected fundraising had built this pioneering new department. A bespoke place to try new experimental methods, test the effects of drugs on leukaemia cells, see if there's a way to change this incurable scourge. They would grow leukaemia cells in enclosed petri dishes, like those from school chemistry classes, to monitor the effects in a controlled environment. Indeed, there was a huge Everest to climb but it seemed, to those standing at base camp looking up, that they had nothing to lose.

And so, this new work began. From the outset they were looking for the origins of the disease, testing new treatments against a background of near total fatality.

Drugs used had been particularly troublesome when dealing with cancer through the years. Either their toxicity, or generally unknown chemical impacts on humans, meant they could certainly kill cancerous cells but they'd bludgeon their way through the body, annihilating lots of good cells in the process. If Hardisty and his peers could find a way to blitz only the cancer cells with chemicals, ignoring healthy cells, they dreamed that they could give children a better outcome than Susan. And there was a particular drug that Hardisty was desperate to trial.

Horror in the Adriatic

There are conflicts throughout history, moments in time, that flare up for a brief period and just as quickly dissipate, committed to the annals of the past. They are no less impactful to those that experience them but are soon forgotten in the collective consciousness. Sometimes there are instances in the long arc of history that impose themselves. Moments of chance, or perhaps perfect design, that ripple far and long from the source.

Such an event occurred in the first week of December 1943 when Lieutenant Colonel Stewart Francis Alexander received a short and unexpected telegram with instructions to travel directly to Bari, Italy. He was to investigate a suspected chemical attack against Allied forces.

Lt. Alexander was an expert in the diagnosis of chemical warfare but, with good reason, hadn't expected to be called into action. As he planned for the journey, he was unaware that the Italian port city on the Adriatic Sea resembled a *Dantesque* vision of hell.

On the night of 2nd December, with the harbour full to capacity hosting British, Norwegian, American and Italian ships, 105 German Luftwaffe planes launched a surprise bombardment from skies overhead. For over 20-minutes relentless explosions rained down, catching the Allies cold. The scene was the stuff of nightmares. Blasts flung sailors overboard, ripped bodies apart or torched them, fires took hold, sirens wailed and wretched screams - *"accents of anger, voices deep and hoarse"* - echoed around the bay. Anti-aircraft gunners shot skyward in desperation, lighting the night like a firework display, as ships burned. Human tissue is delicate. Smouldering jagged shrapnel tore flesh in all directions, blood pools rose in the water, dense black smoke whipped and billowed from sunken holes where decks used to be. *"Round through that air with solid darkness stain'd"*[cxii].

The attack was over but the terror just beginning.

Dock workers and sailors alike found themselves plunged in the water, no recollection of how they landed there, displaced from land or vessel by a blast they didn't see coming. Flames angrily roared from each of the British and American frigates hit, fuelled by the oil and cargo they carried onboard, all of which now gushed through open cavities into the water below. Coating the surface, oil covered water was on fire. Soldiers swam searching safety, dragging with them grease-coated comrades from the wrecks or watching on as those trapped beyond reach roasted alive in a furious inferno. In war soldiers are no longer children, but they are someone's child.

The heat was unbearable. Many fires independently blazed, feeding on plentiful materials at their disposal. Local citizens looked on from afar, the stench of burning oil filling their nostrils. Rescue teams continued in the waters until they realised, quite suddenly, that they needed to retreat. From the hull of a nearby vessel, they heard hissing. *"A groaning sound, and hisses with the wind. That forces out its way, so burst at once."* When a container filled with combustible material reaches certain temperatures, and pressure builds with nowhere to go, an exothermic reaction takes place releasing a sudden and violent release of energy. For the 40 ships ablaze in Bari harbour that night they were no longer boats fuelled and prepped for battle. They were bombs.

Erupting in a domino effect the battlecruisers, moored side-by-side, exploded in-turn, each a catalyst for the next. These were monumental blasts anew. The last to blow, and the biggest of the lot, was the SS John Harvey, a 440-foot US cargo ship whose explosion lit up the night sky. It left behind an evil ditch, *"With flames so numerous throughout its space, Shone the eighth chasm, apparent"*. Each new blast fired razor sharp sizzling metal off at all angles, flames ripping across trails of surface oil and each, in turn, thrusting a canon of water a mile high into the sky, returning as a monumental torrent to pound all below.

As the sun rose on 3rd December, Bari harbour was in ruins and over 1,000 people dead. Sailors took small boats out into the gloopy waters, prodding through the oil and debris in recover torn-up body parts floating near the surface. The air was sombre. *"Then sorrow seized me that e'en now revives, As my thought turns again to what I saw."*

The local hospital was filled with those injured as medics bandaged and fixed all they could. As the hours passed new patients turned up at the hospital desperately seeking help but their symptoms were peculiar. Many showed blisters, the size of balloons, bulging from their skin, dermatitis, lesions or burn marks, despite claiming they'd escaped injury in the blast. Some suffered severe breathing issues, sight loss with eyes swollen shut and uncontrollable vomiting. Others even had painful elephantiasis of the genitalia. Hospital staff had no clue. Some of the patients didn't have even a scratch on their bodies. But one-by-one their skin would blotch and start turning brown. They'd be sat up in their bed chatting away and then, moments later, they'd collapse and die.

Rumours began to spread. Had the Germans used chemical weapons when bombing the port? After the use of mustard gas in World War I, which killed over 90,000 on all sides, the 1925 Geneva Protocol banned the use of chemical and biological weapons in warfare[xxiii]. It was recognition that some weapons were too horrible, even for war. If the Nazis used poisonous gas, it would constitute a war crime. But witnesses hadn't smelt garlic, the odour of mustard gas, so there had been no suggestion of foul play.

As the death toll continued to rise over the following days from unknown causes, General Eisenhower sent for Dr Stewart Alexander; the foremost expert on chemical weapons that the US had.

Alexander's first stop was the Bari General Hospital to see the victims himself. On the ward beds Navy men exhibited the mysterious symptoms, complaining of skin sores, vision loss and nausea. He visited the basement; a 75-foot-long dark corridor, no more than 8-feet wide, cold and without lights; his torch revealed bodies laid out lengthways, one after the next, all of whom had died in the days *after* the bombing. He went to the port, inspected the burnt-out carcasses of ships, watched as locals scooped a layer of oily slime from the water surface.

It took Alexander no time at all to determine the cause; mustard gas. Without question. He'd worked at Edgewood Arsenal, Maryland for many years, conducting tests and experiments using mustard gas and he knew the indicators better than anyone. He also knew the chemical hadn't been dropped in a bomb by the Germans, the injuries were markedly different when inhaled. Although official records begged to differ, it must have been stored on, and released from, a cargo ship in the harbour. He deduced that the chemical agent had been onboard the John Harvey.

His claim was immediately denied outright by his superiors in the US Navy while the British refused to release information. In reality, when the SS John Harvey had left its home at Wilminton, North Carolina in August, she had been storing 2,000 mustard bombs in her hold. Despite only intended in a retaliatory capacity, the storage of chemical weapons in a warzone was a breach of the protocol, nonetheless. As the liquid mustard was released into the waters, all sailors and dock workers swimming for safety were exposed to its dangers[xxiv].

Dr Alexander's initial report showed that the mustard gas had severely impacted the formation of new white blood cells in the patients he studied. It totally stunted the stem cells' ability to reproduce immune defences – it stopped them multiplying - and left the individual powerless against viral attack. But his written report was censored and suppressed by the Allied forces. They feared knowledge of this would embolden the Nazis to use the chemical warfare agent in retaliation.

In Germany, Joseph Goebbels, the Reichsminister of Public Enlightenment and Propaganda, heralded the attack as a stroke of tactical genius – the biggest aerial attack in the Mediterranean - and a resounding success. He didn't, however, make reference to any chemical agent. Nor were they aware soldiers were dying for any reason other than the bombs. At the beginning of the war, British Prime Minister, Winston Churchill, was resolute that Britain would not use mustard gas. That is, unless the German's used it first. In which case all bets were off. It was a reciprocity clause written into the Geneva Protocol, which also applied to the Germans, that if chemical agents were used in warfare the opposing forces would be free to do the same. Of course, the Nazis used chemical agents in another harrowingly genocidal way during World War II, away from the battlefield in the gas chambers of concentration camps, violating much more than just the Geneva Protocol.

Alexander's report may have been silenced but, as more patients arrived seeking help from the effects, his insight guided the medics in the hospital to effectively treat for mustard gas exposure. While no one outside of Bari knew it until decades later when the papers were declassified, Alexander's diagnosis and action saved numerous lives. Dr Stewart Alexander suspected, however, he may have landed on something bigger. His observations at the port in Bari had demonstrated mustard's suppressive effect on cell division. He hypothesised this could be used to inhibit the fast-multiplying malignant white cells that can invade and destroy healthy tissue. It could be used to slow down cancer.

After the war, Stewart Alexander and his well-connected boss took the report to General Motors (GM) tycoons, Alfred Sloan and Charles Kettering, with a request to fund a new state-of-the-art laboratory to develop treatment for cancer. GM may have felt they had some making up to do. Their facilities in Germany had offered industrial production of trucks, torpedoes, land mines and Luftwaffe aircraft throughout the war. Their business may have even contributed to the planes that bombed Bari harbour that night. Not that it troubled them much. Sloan was quoted as telling shareholders that the manner in which the Nazi government ran Germany "should not be considered the business of the management of General Motors"[xxv]. Nevertheless, the funding was agreed, and the Sloan Kettering Institute for Cancer Research (SKI) was established. The first order of business was to develop new synthesised mustard derivatives and grow this medicine to treat cancer. The drug they produced is known today as chemotherapy. Due to the Bari bombing, the age of cancer chemotherapy was born.

A balancing act of chemicals

Incorporating chemical chemotherapy into treatment was key to Roger Hardisty at the Hospital for Sick Children at Great Ormond Street. He wanted to use it as part of a treatment for leukaemia, dialling down the growth of cancerous cells for long enough that other interventions, such as fresh bone marrow, could get to work. It didn't start well. The centre, with the donations of the Leukaemia Research Fund (which is now, a few name-changes later, Blood Cancer UK) set up by the Eastwood's, introduced chemotherapy and steroid solutions initially. It was a little rough-and-ready. Even in encouraging cases, where drugs had slowed the growth of cancerous cells and the child had entered remission, there was still little hope of a full recovery. If the drugs were stopped, the cancer would come back, along with symptoms such as bone marrow failure, anaemia and bleeding. Dosages were not yet refined either and, even when leukaemia cells were shrunken or killed, many children died of common infections due to the damage the drugs had inflicted on their bodies[xxvi].

By the early 1970s, the trials began to pay off. Pioneering a new approach to chemotherapy, including exciting drug combinations and tweaks to dosages[xxvii], was delivering promising outcomes. A 1971 study highlighted how long-term survival for children with acute leukaemia treated at Great Ormond Street had trebled since 1963[xxviii]. Dr Hardisty and his team were finally ascending their Everest climb; something once considered impossible, now seeing increasing success.

It was time for a national trial and, partnering with other microbiology experts. Hardisty focused on acute lymphoblastic leukaemia (ALL), the most common form of childhood cancer. They combined two main aims: killing cancer cells and shrinking tumours. Both options were without too much finesse or evidence but this was what trials were all about. As well as pumping the children's bodies with chemicals, those selected for the trial would be blasted with high doses of radiation. Neither scientific art form was gentle, nor were they the finished article, but for the first time saw the adoption of combining early radiotherapy with a treatment of chemotherapy. The results saw dramatic impacts on survival rates. Pretty soon, the technique was rolled out across paediatric cancer care across the UK.

Dr Hardisty, who was open – and a little desperate – to try something new was the first specialist to be solely concerned with paediatric haematology in Britain and his colleagues started down a path that would transform the outcomes for children, and adults, with cancer. His influence on paediatric treatment to this day is tangible and his impact between 1960-1980, against a backdrop of catastrophic failure, is epic. By the time he stepped away from Great Ormond Street in 1987, he'd helped to transform the 100% death rate for children with leukaemia in the 1950s to a staggering 70% survival rate[xxix].

A key component to this success was his introduction of lower intensity chemotherapy treatment paired with radiation for children. It targeted the immune system in a more delicate way, supressing the growth of cancerous cells and allowing the young patients to benefit fully from the other aspects of treatment. Seen by experts across the world, his approach to chemotherapy in treating blood disease was widely emulated.

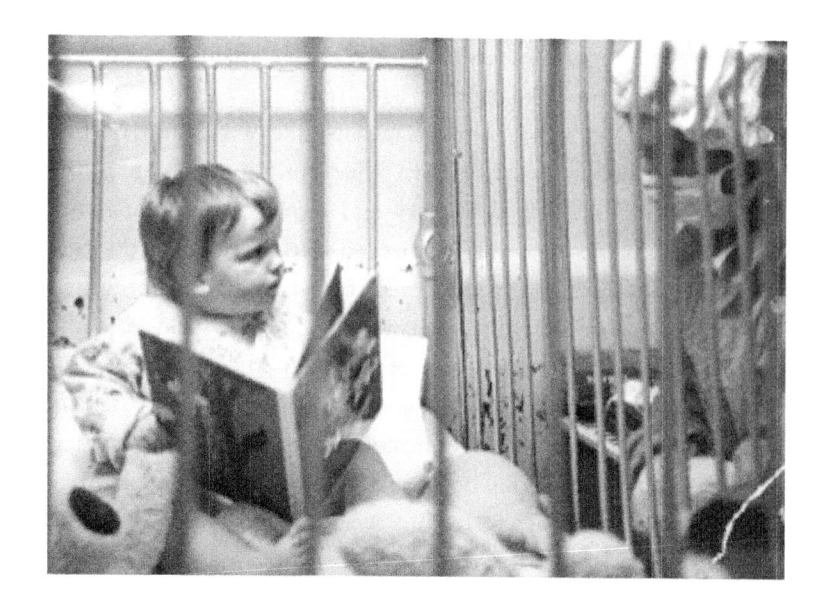

On the eve of transplant
12th April, 1973

Engulfed by the relative comfort of the green parent dorms, Liz's night hours were fitful. Cosily enclosed in the calm parental quarters on the top floor, she felt warm but trapped. Through the rain kissed glass of the bowed window, silhouettes of tree branches grabbed like elongated fingers tapping at angles, not pausing for a moment. They rattled against a backdrop of an azure city lit sky.

Everyone beyond the green room was asleep, resting. But Liz could not. As she lay in bed, a flurry of fast rushing footsteps brushed and scuffed just beyond the door; a vivid memory of when she occupied this room the night Andrew died. The nervous pause as the feet beyond came to a halt, dappled light from the corridor seeping through the gap, before raptures against the wood and hurried heartbeats, cradling her first-born child for the final time. She couldn't rest here. The flashbacks and terrors that haunted her nights lived in this room. They dwelled in the depths of the jade carpet; seeped through the shadowed striped wallpaper, permeated the fusty air. Not the vibrant shamrock tones of spring but the deepest of seaweed green, of tree leaves in the late throws of Autumn. Life draining, darkness and despair impatient to step in. They didn't want her to forget, jealous plausibly of her chance at maternal redemption. This boy could survive. Very soon she may never see this room again, feel it's weighted judgement, hear the flustered scurry of feet approach.

Each restless night was followed by an agitated day. This her sixth in succession in the Victorian turret, fastened to the corner of the old Westminster Children's Hospital. As she lay awake, she'd recall a nurse once telling her that this section of the building had been ripped off during the war; an explosion from a bomb dropped during the Blitz – around the same time as the Bari air raid - partially destroying the lower floors. The building, known back then as the Infants Hospital, continued to function as much of London did during those years. Liz found it strangely comforting to think that, even before she was born, this building was still a place of caring for the capital's sick children. They must know what they were doing by now. As the night hours intensified the troubles inside her mind, she thought back to the commotion she'd caused the previous evening. Angered by unsterile and even dirty conditions on the ward, she'd ripped up the transplant consent forms and thrown them aside. Staff laziness risked her Simon's life. The procedure could not go ahead without them.

A few hours later, she received the phone call behind the bar of The Royal Oak, passed the three or four or more reporters waiting for the family having walked through the rain soaked square. Was she making the right decision? Soot and dust and dead insects covered the tiled corridors. She saw them ever-present in her mind's eye, taunting her. Was she the only one that could see them? Were they really even there or was obsession clouding her perception?

Her mind felt crowded. Unsure of distinction between reality and the intermediary state you exist in before sleep. More hurried footsteps beyond the bedroom door. Loud this time, urgent. She turned her head ever so slightly. No one was there.

Her husband, Roger, lay undisturbed in the other single bed a few feet away. He was always so tired, ongoing treatment for his own hidden predator left him exhausted each day. She observed him breathing for a few seconds, the steady rise and fall of his chest a calming rhythm for her own inhalations to emulate. Roger was always by her side, a gentle and reassuring beat to contrast her periodic mania. She accepted that she could sometimes be a little difficult, perhaps even troubled, but that their partnership was a delicate balance always. Onlookers, like Mollie, may view Roger as a meek man: a timid and docile guy who whimsically unfurled and recoiled from one day to the next without purpose or drive. Liz believed he could be more than that. His fire wasn't snuffed out just yet. But he was still sick, left scrawny from the treatment and even a little yellow in some lights. A shadow of the man she married, troubled by the cancer, privately grieving the death of his son.

Liz had metamorphosised more times than a moth: from new wife to new mother; from new mother to patient mother; to primary carer to grieving parent; and then back to the role of caregiver. Not just for her child but also for her husband. The plight of a main caregiver is that they always feel the need to care more. Their work is never done. She was fulfilling what she believed to be her primary purpose as a woman, the absolute peak of femininity. To raise children, she believed, was why she was born. Wasn't that the sign of ultimate womanhood?

Liz focused her gaze on the flitting branches reaching towards the roof, wincing each time they clattered against the glass. She had never thought twice about her life choices; she'd known her purpose from a young age was to be a mother. It had allowed her the freedom to put less pressure on her chosen job, to clock in and out as required to build-up to a rewarding role as parent. But, after the death of Andrew and now Simon's perilous condition, she allowed her mind to wander. Her upbringing had very much focused on a woman's place being in the home. Similarly, Roger's upbringing echoed that focus on a father 'bringing home the bacon'. There was something comfortable about it, for Liz. Something uniform and relaxed; she knew where she stood.

As the world changed around her, slowly but meaningfully, perhaps she wondered if she could have been part of it. Women factory workers in Dagenham had gone on strike demanding the same pay as the blokes and the Equal Pay Act came about as a result. All women in England, Scotland and Wales could now access the contraceptive pill after campaigning, rather than it being only married women when their husbands 'allowed' it. The UK's first women's refuge opened its doors in Chiswick supporting victims of domestic violence.

Inspiring women were breaking boundaries and challenging the structured order. Maybe Liz wondered if she was doing enough. Perhaps these changes gave her confidence to sign the exclusive contract with the Daily Express. She could use her column to tell her family's story, build awareness and raise vital funds for children to have life-saving treatment. A regular newspaper feature could achieve all that. Liz pledged her allegiance to them. The Westminster Children's Hospital didn't have enough equipment, didn't have enough plastic bubbles, didn't have enough staff. She had a profile now, some small degree of fame. This would be her way to make her mark. Was *she* becoming a campaigner?

She'd perhaps subscribed unwittingly to the narrative of her peers and of the time. Women, overall, were not to focus on education, careers and politics but on homemaking, childbearing and motherhood. This green room where she lay was named 'The Mothers Quarters', where doting mothers stayed and rested during visits. Or *tried* to rest. Fathers were allowed, of course, but woman were perceived to be the caring ones. Her church spoke of a woman's biological role, their lesser involvement in organised religion and matrimony being about pledging to submit and obey. This was her way to navigate that complex landscape. She certainly didn't require motivating.

Laying transfixed in a state of non-sleep, Elisabeth recalled the episode the previous night with nervous dread. She'd shouted and screamed and ripped up the order of play. Not bad for a subjugated woman that would amount to nothing. Liz was persistent, a little rash in her decisions sometimes, but definitely someone you'd rather have on your team than in opposition. She was a little anxious - unrepentant but wondering whether she had upset the doctors and staff. They were mostly men, the senior staff at least. Photos on the walls of the hospital showed that Board of Directors were also all men. She felt surrounded. The men were making all the decisions about the future of the mother's babies. Maybe the episode was her way to take back a bit of control. Simon was *her* son, after all.

Her eyes were closed now but she was still awake, thinking. Where was the donor right now? Was she sleeping? She'd arrived earlier that day. Of all the hundreds and thousands of people that had responded to the newspaper appeal she was just thankful one of them – this incredible person nearby – was a match for her Simon. While the others may not have the right blood this time, perhaps one day they will get the chance to save another. By testing all these people, by cataloguing the diversity of a population, perhaps some of them will be given that incredible opportunity. What if this list of people continued to grow over the months and years? Would the chances of a match for the next child, and the next, and the next get better every time the catalogue expanded. With the transplant planned for tomorrow (or maybe it was now in fact today, as the hours lagged on), she must be sleeping somewhere nearby. Liz devoted her faith to this stranger. She pictured her asleep and comfortable; a thought that finally brought Liz some inner quiet.

A health service for all
1972/73

Flattening the dark blue creases of her dress flush to her leg, Caroline lowered herself onto the wall, close attention fixed on the steaming mug of black coffee swilling close to the edges in her other hand. She couldn't afford to spill a drop of it today. Still standing but circling restlessly nearby Mira savoured the last drags of her cigarette. The fourth of the shift.

Her head pounded with incessant bother as she stamped out the stick and took up her space on the wall next to her colleague. Curling the woollen coat collar up to cover her neck from the chill, she cosied up close and interlocked Caroline's arm with her own to share warmth.

The duo of junior doctors sipped in silence for a minute or two, watching from their vantage point through a cloud of visible breath as children galloped across the grassy square in front of them; let out from school and bulldozing their way home for dinner. Still at last. Fatigue resurfaced again after a spell of dormancy; a spectre rising to torment from the ground, grasping at limbs, tugging down greedily with a heavy weight. Without the caffeine they'd surely be done for, overwhelmed.

It wasn't the only drug that kept them going. Adrenaline had them relentlessly toiling around the clock, the clear need for their skill a catalyst for their renewed energy. The shift pattern was brutal. A 24-hour day and night shift over a 12-day rota. They lived on the job, slept at the job. The miles they padded, the fleeting respite they seized. These quiet minutes were savoured.

"I told the father that if he feels strongly about his daughter not being treated by nurse Kathleen, he could go to find lifesaving treatment elsewhere. He knows full-well that he doesn't have the benefit of choice."

Mira's tone was sharp, her lips thin. Caroline had been at the other end of the ward when she'd heard raised voices coming from some of the parents. As she'd rounded the corner and saw the commotion her heart sank, immediately recognising what her colleagues were dealing with.

Caroline could still visualise the stunned faces of the children. Their heads tilted in the direction of the scene, silently motioning to follow their gaze. A mother tepidly tugged her husband's sweater as he gesticulated with an extended index finger to Mira and Professor Hobbs. The worst of it seemed to have passed. Hobbs was subduing the little girl's father, palm extended placatingly. Mira stood by his side, a delicate balance of physical restraint and facial rage.

Behind Mira, in the doorway of the nursing office, Kathleen watched on with a look of embarrassed indignity. As Caroline approached the scene through the central walkway between bed ends, Kathleen's gaze switched in her direction to reveal water that filled her eyes balancing on the precipice. She cradled her hands around her midriff, scared to blink and release cascading tears, comforting herself as others fought in her honour. In a single sweeping motion Caroline engulfed, spun and seated Kathleen in the private staff office. Eyes closed, and without crying, tears fell.

There was no need for questions. Caroline knew what had happened despite arriving late to the scene. Ward Sister's at other hospitals may turn a blind eye to instances of racism, but not here. Short of a punch in the face, the ferocity of the response made it unquestionably clear to the father that objection meant ejection. A hand on Kathleen's knee, Caroline simply showed her silent support, allowing the hurt to pass and composure return.

In need of help

When learning about the treatment of blood disease in the UK, and the creation of a stem cell transplant register, it's important to recognise the context in which it all played out. Unlike most countries around the world at the time, research and treatment took place in a unique system that provided universal healthcare.

When the National Health Service (NHS) was launched in Britain in 1948 it brought with it an enticing promise of free healthcare for all. Those needing bone marrow transplants, or indeed any British citizen in sick health, could now turn to this service to help them get well again.

In the wake of World War II, the electorate had decided to vote out their wartime leader, Winston Churchill, replacing him with Labour Party candidate, Clement Atlee. A key aim of the party had been a form of socialised medicine, equitably free at the point of need to all Britons, regardless of wealth. Spearheading this bold policy, which would involve nationalising over 2,500 hospitals, was the new Minister of Health, Aneurin (Nye) Bevan. The Welshman used the membership model of the Tredegar Medical Aid Society, based in his hometown, to design the NHS. The welfare state wasn't a simple tick-box exercise for the Labour Government though and Bevan faced opposition from those outside and inside his own party. Churchill's Conservative Party had voted against launching an NHS

21 times believing it to be the "first step to turn Britain into a National Socialist economy".

The greatest barrier, however, came from the British Medical Association, who called Bevan "a complete and uncontrollable dictator", dramatically arguing that, as in Germany, the Minister for Health would become a "medical Fuhrer[xxx]". There was plenty of unrest among doctors and consultants themselves too. The general mood focused on the fear that this new nationalised approach would limit their ability to see, and charge, private patients. Desperate not to let the grand plan fall short, concessions were made and Bevan claimed he'd been forced to pay them off, stating, "I stuffed their mouths with gold" to secure the support of GPs.

As Bevan opened the doors of the National Health Service (NHS) it coincided, almost exactly, with Britain opening its doors to newcomers in the post-war mass movement of once-colonial populations from the, so-called, 'New Commonwealth'.

HMT Empire Windrush landed at a misty Tilbury Docks, Essex, on 21 June 1948. Setting off from Trinidad in May, the ship had picked up passengers in Jamaica, Mexico, Cuba and Bermuda before concluding its journey docking on the English south coast. The following day, Tuesday 22nd June, 1,027 energised and optimistic passengers disembarked to begin their new life, overtly encouraged by the British government to cross the Atlantic to the 'mother country' by job opportunities amid the UK's post-war labour shortage. While still jubilant in the wake of victory in the war, the country was very much on its knees. It found itself in desperate need of imported labour to work at every level, and in almost every industry, to help rebuild Britain from scratch. For some it was felt undesirable to have non-white workers but the need for recovery left no alternative. Over half of those onboard that first ship were

Jamaican, and Calypso bands played on the deck throughout the arduous two-month journey, entertaining passengers travelling from elsewhere in the Caribbean, Polish nationals displaced during the conflict and other Britons returning home from military service.

A few weeks later, on 5th July, Bevan was handed the keys to the Park Hospital in Trafford, Manchester; a symbolic moment to launch a free health service based on "pure Socialism and as such opposed to the hedonism of capitalist society". From day one, the NHS used intentionally inclusive language in all pamphlets and propaganda to get the message to the population that this was 'your' NHS and that it was available to everyone: 'rich or poor, man, woman or child'. The rhetoric focused on "equalitarianism", a term explicitly used to define the NHS in contemporary press at the time. Official portrayals of the NHS, however, painted a somewhat different picture. When it came to photos, cartoons and promotional material, the NHS consistently depicted the vulnerable and deserving patients of the service as white people. Early newsreels covering the NHS likewise showed a service uniformly provided by, and to, the white majority community. Throughout the period of Empire there were minority ethnic groups in Britain but relatively low in number. By 1951, those who had been born in the New Commonwealth and Pakistan living in Britain was estimated to be 256,000, doubling to around 500,000 by 1961. Those British subjects disembarking the Empire Windrush that day in June 1948, and subsequent arrivals and next of kin, were immediately eligible to receive all NHS services.

There was a rumbling anxiety and fear among some media and the populous about the newcomers accessing 'their' health service. Just three-months after the 'NHS Appointed Day' in June, people protested about 'medical tourism' and, within the year, there were parliamentary debates about foreigners abusing 'our' NHS, entering

Britain solely to benefit from free healthcare. A few months later, debates changed focus talking of the 'burdensome and undeserving immigrants' taking up much needed beds and the increasing visibility of 'foreign' doctors.

'Race' was the dominant term used in post-war Britain to explain the presumed and perceived human differences between recently arrived populations (and sometimes their descendants) and the majority population. 'Colour' and 'coloured' were used as socially acceptable generic terms in discussing population groups who could be visually distinguished by skin tone and hair texture. As the concept of biological race became increasingly untenable, scientifically and politically, 'race' and 'colour' were gradually and partially replaced by 'ethnicity' as the preferred term for categorizing and discussing British populations.

Those foreigners clogging up the system

The post-war mass migration led to the emergence of another debate about the newcomers being dangerous vectors of disease, infectious and scrounging. It's not a new concept; that a sick foreigner will come to our shores bringing infectious disease can be traced back to Victorian Britain and beyond. Bram Stoker's 'Dracula', perhaps the most infamous infected immigrant of all, tapped into the fear of invisible threats finding their way in and dismantling orderly tradition. This became known as the 'coloured problem'; that's not to say all immigrants had black or brown skin but that pigmentation was the most obvious distinction of 'otherness'. More concerning was the supposed or presumed health impacts of mass migration, burdensome and undeserving immigrants, sometimes even strengthened by official sources in Government.

The British Medical Association campaigned vocally and vigorously to have all new entrants to the UK medically screened. Further fuelling the 'infectious immigrants' image, radiographic screening was set up at Heathrow Airport in 1964 on the lookout for tuberculosis, disproportionately stopping non-white travellers. But when the TV channels broadcast the scramble for vaccinations after an outbreak of smallpox there were very rarely non-white faces 'clogging up' the system.

There seemed to be a difficulty understanding these new and unfamiliar names at first. Many patients received the wrong medication, confusion in the records meant regular mix-ups with appointments and prescriptions. Staff struggled to differentiate their Chowdhury's from their Chakrabarti's or their Kumbhar's from their Kumar's. The overseeing Ministry of Health observed from a distance but offered no formal guidance, electing not to influence the fledgling NHS service in action.

Paradoxically, some of those non-white workers became symbols of care and cure, saviours of the fragile and nascent NHS itself, and of its dependence on imported labour. Increased access to television news no longer obscured the diversity of staff: medical saviours from all corners of West India, Africa and Asia. And not simply in operating theatres or nursing the sick. Without the porters, carpenters and other non-medical workers the whole thing wouldn't have got off the ground.

After the Notting Hill riots in 1958, tabloid cartoonists depicted racist skinheads as the butt of the jokes, ironically turning up to be treated for their injuries by non-white medical teams. Yet still no photographs of these doctors or nurses appeared in NHS marketing material. Tempered by the public mood the service itself somewhat ignored their reliance on non-white professionals.

We'll learn more about these health inequalities, and potential explanations, a little later in the book. While there was little visual evidence to support arguments of burdensome immigrant patients, the 20 post-war years saw increasing media coverage of the optically striking diversity among its staff. Irish and Caribbean nurses were integral to the expansion of the NHS in the 1950s and 1960s, and treatment was fundamentally reliant on doctors born and trained overseas.

The Indo-Pakistani War of 1965, however, led a Ministry of Health official to raise concerns that the NHS could be weeks from collapse stating that the conflict "might result in the recall to India and Pakistan of doctors from British hospitals which could therefore face paralysis within weeks". That may have had something to do with a concerted effort to finally acclimatise immigrants to their new surroundings and that same year the BBC launched a radio and TV show called 'Make Yourself at Home', hosted by an Indian-Muslim and spoken in "Hindustani", described by the BBC as a "mixture of simple Hindi and simple Urdu". The key aim was "to help in integration, not assimilation" but this theme didn't seem to transcend into the workplace.

An unspoken skin-tone hierarchy prevailed through the sterile corridors of the health service. Certain nursing roles were more coveted that others and in those early days you'd be unlikely to see a black or brown skinned nurse working in paediatrics, for example. Those desirable roles were reserved for the white nurses leaving the 'others' to asylums and caring for the elderly or infirm. The trend allocated roles to 'newcomers' that were unworthy of the attention of the indigenous population. Teaching Hospitals were a particularly tough nut to crack and were much whiter than non-teaching hospitals across London and the wider country. Colour-barring seemed to exist when it came to the top jobs making it easier to start your own business, a GP practice for example, than to attempt progression in a very white NHS, so many doctors of colour did just that.

Back to work

Things were changing, slowly, but any progress achieved made incidents on the ward taste more bitter.

Caroline drained the final lukewarm sips of coffee from her mug. The mother and grandmother of a young patient smiled as they walked past their seated position on the perimeter wall. A few days prior that grandmother had explained to Kathleen, with no malice or motive, that she was the first Black person that she had ever met. The family were visiting from Newcastle while their son received treatment at the hospital. All the siblings would need to be tested as potential matches so visiting, in instances like this, would often last for many weeks moving the whole family to the capital, at great expense. The parents, bereft of ideas or choice, were investing life savings in the hope of salvation. It was a lot of pressure on the hospital staff.

Caroline had allowed a heavy black tar to coat her heart, trapping within its sticky gloop any pain that tried to get in. It was the only way to weather the blame. This job hadn't made her hard though. She felt the loss in private moments. In order to continually do her best for the patients in her care she was forced to move on, to recharge her belief in their practice, despite the fatal setbacks. Watching a child deteriorate before her eyes, while the eyes of the family despairingly looked to her for answers, would never be easy.

Mira had started to shiver, a sign that their 15-minutes were likely up. They rose in unison, still tightly connecting arms, and made their way back to the main hospital entrance on Udall Street. For every instance when a patient, or parent, refused treatment from a Black doctor or nurse, there were 100 instances quite the opposite. But on each occasion, like when a teacher scolds a classroom for the insolence of a few, it takes some time for the atmospheric build-up to dissipate.

Zipping between beds, a smile radiating to each onlooking child, Kathleen was back at work: taking bloods, checking vitals, keeping the ward operational. The children loved to laugh and joke with her as she completed the rounds. She seemed to convert negativity into something regenerative, soaking up energy and smiles to recharge her power. She didn't accept the comments as part of her job. She didn't absolve remarks like those of the little girl's father. But she decided she had to just get on with it. Her drive and purpose focused acutely on the children. She'd be side-tracked by no bigot.

The undercurrent that blighted the bone marrow transplantation unit on a day-to-day basis in 1972 was less racial and more territorial. As Caroline and Mira hooked their jackets and scarves up on the wall of the staff room in the basement, Jack Hobbs stormed passed the door, disconcertingly mumbling to himself as he went. His language turned the air. You could sense when he was working on something big, something showstopping. They wondered which idea he'd flit to today. He made no bones about his leadership in the department and that only *he* was grabbing pioneering solutions by the scruff of the neck. For his colleagues, often dragged along, the dubious methodology led to vicious feuds that were reaching a fever pitch.

Alright, Jack

Jack is a pivotal character in our history of the bone marrow transplant register. He balanced a bombastically buccaneering style alongside a deep-seated empathy for those facing injustice and life-limiting illness. A relatively tall man, Jack had a lithe physique, with short wavy black hair efficiently combed over and a look in his eyes that showed he was never quite satisfied. He desperately wanted to lead change and he'd haul people down his path, dutifully or otherwise.

His forceful mentality was thought to have come from his upbringing in the military. Born in Aldershot in 1929, his early years were somewhat peripatetic due to his father Frederick's postings as a captain in the Army. Along with his mother Anna and three brothers, Jack travelled around a lot until the family settled in Plymouth, aside from a few years of evacuation to Penzance during the Blitz.

At 16, Jack left school and got straight to work. From a young age he'd been intrigued by nature. Starting out by building his own ant farm, Jack progressed to learning more about the human body often asking teachers troublesome questions in class. He tried to wrap his head around how all these functions can simultaneously be taking place so perfectly and without much input as we go about our daily lives. It stands to reason, then, that his first job out of school was as a pathology lab assistant, focused on body tissue and understanding disease.

Two years later he enlisted for his National Service with the Royal Army Medical Corps (RAMC), ending up in Egypt and Palestine and, on returning, was fully decided on his career path. In 1950 he received a state scholarship to study medicine at the Middlesex Hospital Medical School and, by the time he graduated in 1956, had amassed seven prizes, revealing what his tutors noted as a lively and intelligent approach to his subject. He buttered his bread for a few years doing house jobs at various London hospitals, including the Middlesex, Brompton and Royal Free, but it wasn't long before a life-long love affair with the Westminster Children's Hospital began, stepping through the door as a registrar in 1959. First to welcome him into the world of paediatrics was the hospital's lead haematologist, Professor Joe Humble.

It would later reveal itself as a crucially defining moment for the young graduate and a meeting of minds took place, unusually, in a chapel.

Nottinghamshire-born, Joseph Graeme Humble, was a stalwart of the Westminster Hospital, joining as a 21-year-old medical student in 1934. A large-framed man with dark, wavy hair combed over in a side parting, Joe dressed for the position he aspired to from the very beginning. He spoke with perfect Queen's English, soft yet forceful, and his public speaking was accompanied by a slight hesitancy; not nerves or insecurities but discomfort when compared to conversations with colleagues or patients.

Starting as house physician to the children's department upon qualifying, he moved into pathology and haematology where he'd remain for the next 41-years. He went on to become a crucial individual in the story of bone marrow transplantation and, by the mid-1950s, he'd uncovered pioneering techniques for extracting and infusing marrow, both of which involved large or daunting needles. His advancement had been made possible by his Westminster colleague, D.E. Pegg, who'd discovered a way to preserve extracted marrow for longer through cryopreservation or freezing. Essentially, they could now put the marrow on ice. Humble's life revolved around bone marrow transplantation, but he was hitting a brick wall when it came to survival rates for children. He knew the department, for which he was now responsible, needed fresh ideas.

The logistics of a bone marrow transplantation are a bit like sorcery. Once stem cells have been extracted from a donor and filtered to remove clumps, they are fed directly into the veins of a patient's arm (a bit like being hooked up to an IV drip). Over the course of a few hours this new blood pumps into the circulatory system but it's of no use just staying there. It must navigate its way to the precise place it's needed, deep inside the bone marrow, where it can start making fresh blood. There's no Satnav or pre-programmed instructions so these cells flow along in the gloop, scouting out where a vacancy exists that would benefit from its skills. Once they identify a gap, where existing stem cells aren't working, they step in and get to work.

Inviting the junior physician on a tour of the hospital, Humble had heard good things about the young registrar from counterparts across the city. After starting out in the Children's Hospital, the tour swiftly made the journey over to Horseferry Road where the main Westminster Hospital was located. A few stop-offs and introductions later, Joe took Jack to the first-floor chapel ending up beneath a huge stained-glass window, almost reaching floor to ceiling, created in memorial of King George VI. After playing a key role in the King's 1952 operation to remove his left lung, Humble's name appeared at the top of the memorial alongside the rest of the medical and nursing team that operated that day.

The team had been persuaded, against their better judgement, to carry out the operation at Buckingham Palace, rather than the hospital itself. Bizarrely in the days before the operation the surgical staff of Westminster Hospital were troubled to find certain instruments, and anaesthetic apparatus missing without explanation. Totally strange; like the Secret Service were checking on them somehow. Even an operating table went missing from their theatres way up on the seventh floor.

Accounts of the experience impressed Jack Hobbs immensely and it sealed the deal.

By the time he'd thundered to his office and the door slam had reverberated back up the corridor just travelled, the furious Hobbs, now professor of chemical pathology, vowed he'd been slighted for the last time.

As recently as May of that year Hobbs had led a team to achieve the first successful father-to-child bone marrow graft and the year before, in 1971, we've already learned of their UK-first bone marrow transplantation on a 7-month-old baby using a sibling graft. But, to Jack's annoyance, they were all national, rather than global, firsts.

Deep down Hobbs was still frustrated that his counterparts in Seattle had beaten him to it. In fact, it wasn't so much 'deep down' but rather simmering at the surface in plain sight. He was competitive by nature, somewhat hostile with it, and refused to simply play catch-up. In fact, he questioned their judgements given that the patient receiving the ground-breaking first sibling transplant in 1969 died shortly afterwards, an infection resulting from the so-called 'successful' transplant. Of course, he didn't wish for the patient to die but could they really claim that to have been a success when the recipient barely lived beyond recovery?

Jack felt that British contributions to tackling blood disease were being airbrushed by the Americans[xxxi].

People that met Jack were rarely indifferent about him. He was brave in his convictions, revelled in an argument and could be quite harsh to those he didn't feel shared his values. Some were event scared of him but Jack knew what he was doing was important.

To all intents and purposes, Jack Hobbs was leading the team toward something spectacular. Yet, from his perspective, his peers did not seem to share his urgency. In some instances, he was certain they subjugated his every effort to achieve the unthinkable. When the unrelated matched donor was confirmed in the Netherlands just a few days too late for little Andrew Bostic, Jack suspected the regrettable timing was too inconvenient to be true. Why had it taken so long to track this person down? Had calls been missed or messages been passed on too slowly? There were nerves among the medical and nursing team, of course, but as one young child after the next died before their eyes could they not see that something was better than nothing?

Jack stood at the window in his office. His fingers entwined behind his back massaging one another as he looked out toward the spire of St Stephen's Church rising over the rooftops beyond Vincent Square. He had an important meeting scheduled with the MP for Westminster, Christopher Tugendhat, in an hour that he could well do without.

It had been quite the morning. Vocal disagreements with peers, a mounting concern that the specialist leads were dragging their heels, not to mention the dismal distraction of a racist parent wasting his time and shouting-the-odds about sub-standard care. It hadn't been the preparation he'd envisaged. But this meeting was too important to delay. Funding for the bone marrow unit hinged on results and it was yet to be seen if their recent relative successes had persuaded the new Conservative Government, led by Prime Minister Ted Heath, to sustain the crucial spending. Without it they'd be forced to close the whole thing down before they'd really got started. Everything he and Joe Humble had developed, the last bastion of chance for children with immune deficiencies, would surely stutter to a standstill.

He'd host the politician in the beautifully adorned lecture room, speak with him directly under the commemorative plaque and medallion depicting the devotee, Edith Mond. This institution to treat sick infants, built in her memory after her death by overdose, a powerful legacy. Jack would use her story, and these historic visuals, to emphasise the importance of progress.

Boom, blast and ruin
1973

Walking north on the Avenue de la Convention, in the southern suburbs of modern-day Paris, you'd be forgiven for missing the clues about the place it once was. Passing under the swooping curvature of two-storey stoned archways, you'd not immediately realise that the structure you walked through has existed in this spot since the Middle Ages.

A dwelling originally known as Arcoïalum, the "place of the arches", is now Arcueil and the impressively grand aqueduct you passed under carried water to the Roman city of Lutetia, now known as Paris, sometime around 200-300 AD. In the 1600s the aqueduct was further built upon to take water from the Bièvre river directly to the royal residence at Luxemburg Palace. And the reason it has a second layer? An even longer aqueduct, built around 1870, would bring Parisians water from the river Vanne a little further away.

You'll be pleased you noticed it now as you continue up the avenue, graffiti illustrations lining your route on either side. It's easy to tell you're in the metropolitan suburbs. Splashes of aged urine, leaked petrol and ditched trash bags scent the street; local artists tag buildings, lampposts and even trucks if any stay in one place too long. They depict an array of people, politics and lifestyles: a 'Black Lives Matter' fist, a shout-out for politician Marine la Pen, a mural of Nelson Mandela accompanied with African National Congress (ANC) flag or simply their personalised calling-card; artists and taggers painting their neighbourhood in the unmistakeable colours of suburbia.

Progressing north temporary arts are impressive but perhaps not in the realms of the most famous art of this community. Lyonel Feininger's 1911 painting, Carnival in Arcueil, depicts his joyous time spent in the small town. A blast of colour on canvas, elongated and angular bodies, whimsical costumes, and antic behaviour; fantastical characters treading cobbled streets, musical enticement from the mind of the German-American caricaturist, a leading exponent of Expressionism. Soaring over his row of tall, narrow houses is the famous two-storey aqueduct, the one we just passed under, overlooking the street scene below.

The modern graffiti, however, gives a bit of colour to otherwise pallid, non-descript buildings of the neighbourhood. Except you notice that one does stand out. Opposite a grey, seven-floor apartment block, is a rundown looking rectangular building covered in dense and unruly vines clamped to the concealed exterior. Some of the wildlife shows a hint of colour, green and purple blooms at this time of year, yet most appears dead; clinging on regardless, no one seems to care. The place looks abandoned, left to some degree of ruin, almost entirely reclaimed by nature, such is the volume of growth weighing down the walls, they themselves struggling to keep the frame upright. Items are visible inside, resting against walls; your view unhindered as no curtains or shutters obscure the interior.

Oddly, though, a large concrete barrier with electrified barbed wire protects it from the street. Temporary containers are situated within the walled complex, security staff seem to be keeping tabs on the place. Perhaps with so many graffiti artists in town the owners want to avoid urban exploration and creative tagging of this obscure little building. But the heightened security is probably not much needed; it's unlikely trespassers would want to break into this empty property.

Inside is the long-since deserted laboratory of Marie Curie.

In 1911, the year that Feininger painted the scene she could see from her lab window, Curie attended the Royal Swedish Academy of Sciences to become the world's only double Nobel laureate, and still the only person to win the prize in two science disciplines. At the same time she faced a personal scandal; an affair with physicist Paul Langevin, and the wrath of the French press. Wrath of the public too. She and her children were threatened in the street for wrecking the marriage of a younger man. Legendary status in chemistry but her reputation away from the laboratory was somewhat in tatters.

After picking up the prize in Sweden, Curie rented an apartment at 36, Quai de Béthune, on the Ile Saint Louis, in her maiden name, Madame Skłodowska. She wished for some quiet, to just get on with her work, and lived there for the rest of her life. In 1933, after outgrowing her existing workplace, the University of Paris gifted Curie this now abandoned building in a suburb south of the city. She only worked there for one-year, until her death in 1934 aged 66, but in that short time managed to practice sufficient chemistry to make the building one of the most radioactive sites in France to this day.

As the discoverer of radium and polonium (named after her native Poland), Curie very well knew there was danger associated with radiation. After all, she was the 'mother of modern physics'; and coined the phrase 'radioactivity'. But she too became radioactive. For years she would casually carry test tubes of radioactive isotopes in her black lab coat pockets and conduct experiments with no safety measures in place. The damaging effects of handling these gloriously glowing substances were not known at the time. And it caused her death; she succumbed to aplastic anaemia; a blood disease caused by exposure to large amounts of radiation over her lifetime.

And all these years later her body, laid to rest at the Pantheon in Paris, is still radioactive. Equally so her laboratory. Known as 'Chernobyl on the Seine', traces of many radioactive materials exist throughout the building, including a uranium isotope found in Marie's papers, furniture, cookbooks and even plants. We measure radioactivity in half-life; the time it will take for one-half of the atom nuclei to decay, for an elements radioactivity to die away. This particular isotope, found in the items Curie left behind, has a half-life of 4.5 billion years.

Glow sticks

Imagine being present in a moment of great historical significance. If we could step through a photograph of 1933 Arcueil, sit on the pavement, and watch Marie Curie walk up the street to her office, unknowing of the globally famed scientist she would be almost 100 years later.

That same profound feeling of reverence or veneration we experience when we find ourselves in a place of great significance. Standing on the steps of the Lincoln Memorial, looking out over the reflecting pool to the Washington Monument, overwhelmed to stand on the precise spot Martin Luther King Jr delivered his iconic speech. Walking through the gateway arch at Auschwitz; following the footsteps of Nelson Mandela's walk to freedom; or standing below blue plaques placed on buildings across London describing a famous scholar, artist, musician, scientist or other that used to walk, breath the air, look up at the stars, exactly where you are.

Before radioactivity was fully understood, Marie Curie in Arcueil wasn't the only one misguided in a casual approach to radioactive material.

In the 1920s, drinking radium water was believed to be a method of healing for cells and tissues. Water was stored in a 'Revigator'; a uranium and radium-laced ceramic container that people would fill each night before bed, let the irradiation do its thing overnight while you slept, and wake up to drink the tainted liquid with a view to curing everything from arthritis to impotence. The company responsible claimed at the time that "water without radioactivity was like air without oxygen". When people started to drop dead from this 'miracle' water, the connection was made.

Others were adamant on the benefits of adding radioactive material to toothpaste. We all want that glowing smile, right? Companies, including the German brand, Doramad, were quite proud of the results after adding thorium to their ingredients, in an effort to make teeth shine whiter and kill all the unwanted germs.

In 1933 Parisian Dr. Alfred Curie (no relation to Marie or Pierre but hoping his name may increase sales) signed off on a range of skin products under the name of Tho-Radia. These soaps, skin creams and 'beauty milks' claimed the "regularization of the superficial circulation of the blood, the toning up and strengthening of the tissues of the skin, the elimination of fat, and the removal of wrinkles." It was claimed to help the skin glow and, at the time, the product was a huge hit. The products were filled with thorium and radium; no wonder those using them to moisturise their faces were positively glowing. Despite being quite ill herself, and the person that brought radioactive material to life, Marie Curie actively distanced any association with Tho-Radia products.

Science's ability to repurpose radioactivity effectively for productive usage was taking quite a long time. The inquisitive Henri Becquerel, one scientist leading the way for this transition, was a man of fortunate discoveries.

In early 1896 the scientific community, including Becquerel, became fascinated with the recent discovery of a new type of radiation. Wilhelm Conrad Roentgen had found that the Crookes tubes emitted a new kind of invisible ray that was capable of penetrating through black paper. These newly discovered *x-rays* also penetrated the body's soft tissue and Roentgen substantiated this through an image of the bones in his wife's hand; the first evidence of x-ray imaging. The medical community immediately recognized the potential usefulness of this type of radiation.

Becquerel was curious to investigate further. His father was an expert in phosphorescence, when a light is emitted without any type of combustion or heat causing it. He thought this was extremely similar to what he was hearing about these marvellous x-rays, so put his theory to the test.

Henri had been trying to capture the perplexing effects of these salts. He'd place them on photographic plates, wrap them in thick black paper, and expose them to the rays of the sun. When he came back to check, he unwrapped and developed the photographic plate to find that the outlines of the crystals were clearly visible. But then, as is so often the way in Paris, the weather became cloudy and grey and the sunlight vanishing for days. Giving up hope of better weather, on a grey winter's day in March 1896, Henri wrapped everything back up and placed the experiment in a desk drawer. A few days later, ready to test again, Henri opened the draw and, to his utter shock, the photographic plate showed perfectly clear new images of the crystal uranium salts that had sat there. The salts had emitted light onto the photographic plate without the stimulation of sunlight. Or, in fact, any light. He'd discovered that uranium naturally, and continuously, emits invisible radiation – not just when it seems to be glowing[xxxii]. To this day Becquerel (Bq) is the unit for measuring radioactive substances.

News of Rontgen's x-ray discovery in Germany travelled fast around Europe and, merely six-months after he'd published his paper "On A New Kind of Rays" on 28 December 1895, an unexpected experiment was taking place in Lyon, France. Rather than using radiation to penetrate the skin to visualise bones, the method was being adapted as a possible treatment for cancer.

While cancer was very much seen as a disease of the rich at this time, lower class people across the world faced another more frightening and deadly killer in tuberculosis. In the 19th century, tuberculosis killed one in every seven people in Europe and the U.S., and it was particularly deadly for city dwellers. The disease, commonly known then as 'consumption', also carried the ominous title of the white plague. It particularly impacted small children, with state run campaigns encouraging people to "cover up your coughs and sneezes" and mothers to protect their children, "by your intelligent care snatch him from Death's hands[xxxiii]".

Now, to zap cancer

Little was really known in terms of how to stop tuberculosis killing but experts did realise it was caused by bacteria that seemed to spread through exchange of bodily fluid. Yet at the time the casual dispersal of one's own fluid was bizarrely commonplace.

In Lyon, as was the case almost everywhere at the end of the 1800s, it was quite ordinary for people to walk along the sidewalk, or in a town square, and nonchalantly spit. Public spitting was known as 'expectorating' and was so unquestionably mundane that, as tuberculosis continued to scythe through populations, advertising posters appeared on billboards and shop fronts across the city requesting, for public safety, that citizens 'Don't spit on the street', and to 'beware of the careless spitter'. So weak, apparently, was a person's self-control to hold in their spittle that businesses began producing the sputum bottle; a little blue vessel that people would use to collect their spit as they went about their business, only to empty out a days-worth of gob when they arrived home. These popular containers had many other names too, known as cuspidors, spittoons, or simply sputum cups or sputum bottles. The most popular proved to be the Blue Henry; a portable pocket flask made of cobalt-blue glass that could be used to collect this sticky phlegm produced by the irritated lungs of a person suffering from tuberculosis.

Worries about spreading dangerous bacteria at the time is relevant to the story of radiation as that is exactly what Victor Despeignes thought was causing cancer.

It had already been shown, in Lyon as it happens, that these new x-rays could kill bacteria cells and, as Despeignes believed cancer to be a similar type a parasitic cell, in theory it should work at killing that. The thing is he was only a hygienist at the time, working to develop conditions to keep the city clean and its people healthy. Playing around with x-ray and radiation was just a hobby, his paid focus being cleaning up the waterways and latrines of Lyon, recommending key changes the city should adopt. He certainly wasn't someone ordinarily expected to treat a stomach cancer, nor did he show sound rationale regarding how this treatment may cure the disease. Yet that's precisely what he set about doing.

He managed to get his hands on a newfound power tool, that being the Crookes tube, and an incredible source of light projection through his local contacts the Lumière brothers, Auguste and Louis (they manufactured the Cinématographe motion picture system). Through these devices Victor would blast out some x-rays in the direction of the cancer growth, becoming the first person to experiment with radiation as a form of treatment on 4th July 1896. Precise documentation of the processes he carried out are extremely clear: two half-hour treatments administered each day, one in the morning and one in the evening. While his patient died at the end of the month, which wasn't ideal, the hygienist claimed that the tumour had reduced in size by as much as 50%.

Victor Despeignes' biographer, Nicolas Foray from the University of Lyon, suggests he's somewhat of an antihero of radiation; a rogue practitioner playing rather free and easy with the medical ethics and treatment of patients. So too with what he deemed as success, it turns out.

In a very specific way, Despeignes' unconventional experiment set the wheels in motion to transform how medicine practically used this latest science to treat disease. As far as we know, and if we are to believe his claims, he was the first to apply radiotherapy to shrink a tumour.

An increasing number of oncologists began incorporating radiation into their treatment plans for patients with cancer. Perhaps they saw something worth developing in Despeignes' trials. It was rough and ready. Full doses of radiation blasted the target area, and the same again after 14 days, the idea behind the 'saturation method', keeping tissues near their tolerance limit. There were extremely toxic side effects from such large doses of radiation and in the 1930s a new little-and-often fractionation method was introduced, led by Henri Coutard, consisting of lower dose treatment administered more frequently. Coutard believed that the radiosensitivity of the cancer cells was the same as that of the regenerative cells of the tissue of origin. By keeping the dosage low, he could give the tissue time to recover before blasting again.

It worked much better. Coutard's low dose fractionation technique led to adoption by oncologists in Europe and North America over the next 20 years and he was credited with developing radiotherapy into a clinical discipline.

Perfecting the radioactive art

At the time of Simon Bostic's potential transplant in the 1970's, these methods were being developed even further. A pioneer trialled new methods to treat children preparing for bone marrow transplantation.

Positioned just so, a canon-shaped shooter aimed directly at the child stood uneasily at the other end of the long corridor. Ann removed herself from view and initiated the blast. There was no screaming from the young boy, no reaction at all really, as he received faintly reassuring smiles and nods from the other side of a nearby glass door. Albeit a far distance away, the noise rumbled deafeningly along the hall, relentless in its grinding churn. As the 20-minutes progressed alone inside the tunnel, the boy became agitated, initially from boredom and then through fear. His time alone in the cold corridor of the hospital basement lost its appeal.

And then it was over. The boy hadn't felt a thing but was, by now, a little worked up. The nurses returned in a hurry, covered head-to-toe in protective equipment; masks shielded faces, gloves coated hands, a net hid their hair. Yet the young boy could still identify who they were. The crinkles at the edges and the colour of their gaze; their reassuring touch and voices that soothed. They were powerless to take the illness from him but they had a gift to ease the dread.

Wheeled out of sight on a bed, destined for refuge inside a sterile plastic bubble, Ann returned to reset the large, clanging radiotherapy machine. Leaving infants alone in the firing line, with only the incessant booming for company, felt brutal but the alternative was much worse. Full body irradiation, like that just carried out, was the best way to prepare a patient for a bone marrow transplant. To effectively delete an existing immune system, faltering and deadly, in preparation for a new graft of fresh cells to hopefully rebuild from scratch. Tuning the machinery Ann knew her methodology was gifting these children their best shot at recovery. That didn't mean, however, that she enjoyed seeing and hearing their anguish.

This slightly crude technique of full body irradiation was a brand-new method in the UK and Professor Ann Barrett, the expert delivering the crucial radiation rays, the architect.

Specialising in paediatric oncology at the Royal Marden Hospital, Professor Barrett had experimented with Despeignes' blasting and Coutard's fractionation but further honed and perfected techniques. Radiation machines were built to administer the rays in the general direction of the recipient. And the machines were ginormous. Far too large to fit on a normal ward or zap a patient discreetly in the precise spot. Similar to those early computers, with powers immeasurably weaker than handheld smart phones today, the machines were the size of a small room.

For a bone marrow graft to 'take' in a host body the medical team needed to ensure all the existing stem cells, those generating the malfunctioning blood, were dead (or irradiated). With no more faulty blood swimming around, new stem cells, creating the good stuff, had the space to thrive without challenge. Radiation would be used to render existing bone marrow null and void but, to do so across the full body, they'd need a long enough distance for the beam trajectory to hit head to toe. When switched on, the invisible rays would set off from their source outward in a pre-determined direction, travelling through everything in their path. The radiation would penetrate all layers, killing things along the way, totally invisible to the human eye.

At the Royal Marsden the early machine was built by a staffer, Eddie, but no office, ward or contained room offered the required length to suit the trajectory of the radiation. The only feasible option was a seldom used basement corridor, sterile green and white acrylic surfaces lacking warmth or comfort. And so, this is where Ann decided to start delivering the crucial blasts. The patient would stand behind a screen to protect from the full force of the rays but not seeing added to the fear factor. No staff or family were allowed in the room at the time of the radiotherapy, for the obvious risk this posed to their own cells, so the recipient, adult or child, would experience the somewhat traumatic event by themselves.

Leaving a child alone in the room brought challenges. They would lose interest, lose patience or simply cry in fear at what was happening to them so regular breaks were needed to comfort and reassure. Parents and nursing teams would then impotently watch on behind the glass, visible and reassuring but powerless. Hiding tears and their own fears, staff and family were resolute in collective ambition as the whimpering youngster longed for the episode to end.

These treatment sessions would take place on a single day, usually a Saturday, and staff would sit from 9am until 6pm delivering radiotherapy one after the next. After creating trust with families, much of the time was spent supporting them, holistically managing the stress of the situation. But Ann, now a specialist in paediatric care, found this all fantastically exciting. It would be a mistake to consider the working environment one of consistent doom. Yes, the odds of patient survival were intensely poor and medical staff worked day and night in often failed efforts to save children's lives. You'd be forgiven for concluding that mood and morale would be sombre. As it happened they tried to prescribe daily doses of joy and laughter on the wards of the Royal Marsden Hospital, for staff and patients alike. A collective belief in the possibilities, an age of technological advancement and an ever-increasing understanding of methods were upon them to counter the circulatory scourge. Staff backed one another's exploratory ventures, supported each step boldly into the unknown and joyously celebrated the peaks as they came along.

Ann Barrett designed this distinctively new radiology technique; the first full body irradiation technique of its kind in the UK. This approach had never been done before and Ann knew she was pushing the boundaries of what was known to be possible, experimenting and working things out as she went along. The long days, late nights and less than ideal working conditions were manageable. Ann was at the cutting edge of something new. Not that it was without its critics. Radiating children in a cold basement corridor raised eyebrows, both among strangers and colleagues, with many voicing their concerns to shut the practice down. Pioneering new techniques was a rough-and-ready process, requiring not just a little flexibility and, while Professor Ann Barrett treated more and more blood disease children in this intimate setting, she herself was forced to develop a thick skin to repel the attacks from those unwilling to accept new medical developments.

As the door opened down the corridor, Ann glanced up as she continued resetting the machine to see the next young patient walking in, hand-in-hand with his mother. While the Royal Marsden itself specialised in treating leukaemia they often received patients with other immune deficiencies from the nearby Westminster Children's Hospital. Practically speaking the radiotherapy needed was identical so a partnership had been struck between the two hospitals to share patients; they didn't have the in-house expertise of Professor Barrett. This new patient, her third of the morning, had made the journey across town. She grabbed her notes, fashioned a friendly smile and set off in the direction of the new family.

The three-year old boy, wearing orange shorts and a green woolly jumper, giggled with the nurse who distracted his attention. He seemed noticeably weak. His mother's gaze, expectant and hurried, had fixed on Ann from the moment of their arrival. Her dyed-blonde wavy hair framed her face, unruly with flecks of grey yet stylish. She carried off a look of sharp poise, a navy blazer jacket leaving no doubt of her business-like approach, while heavy droops below her eyes cradled hours of restless solitude.

Out of the traps a flurry of questions, abrasive and rough, met Professor Barrett out of the earshot of the young boy. Ann was used to this from family before treatment; to them this was the most crucial treatment she will ever deliver, and she understood that need. This time seemed different, though. This mother showed no signs of fear, but instead battle-ready poise. She seemed weary yet firm; windswept but dogged.

She turned away dismissively to kiss her little lad on the lips, explained she'd be just through the glass, and made tracks for the door. He sat, quite settled, and the nurse moved him to a comfortable position with his toy teddy, itself irradiated before the session. Opening the door to leave the mother turned to look directly at Ann, who'd still not received confirmation that her answers were acceptable. Her furrowed brow softened, just slightly; her lips thinned and a crack at the edge of her mouth inclined to a qualifying smile. Head tilted, her eyes filled, and she left.

Professor Ann Barrett knew that was his mother's way of showing approval. Making her way back up the hallway she knew this was a monumental moment in this family's life; but more than that, what the boy's treatment could mean for the future of bone marrow transplantation. Trajectories double-checked and the initiation sequence in place, Ann left the little boy in the room alone. This specialised radiotherapy a key link in the chain but, like everything, it was experimental. Only time would tell.

New ideas are not to be trusted

"Pain is the mother's safety, it's absence her destruction[xxxiv]."
Sitting at his grand wooden window desk, the private gardens of 52 Queen Street in Edinburgh across the street below, James Young Simpson let out a despondent sigh. In his hand, the latest edition of the Edinburgh Medical and Surgical Journal, in which this quote about pain being a mother's safety glared up at him in print. It was a very public attack, pointed directly at him. His work was under fire, in this widely circulated medical journal, from none other than his own peers. An accusation that his treatment would, if left unchallenged, fundamentally deprive the life of a mother and, perhaps, her baby.
Dismayed, he continued reading. "The blood, robbed by the ether of its oxygen… depreciated as a consequence… intensely blackened… and rendered unfit for the purposes of life."[xxxv]
Philosophically, they argued, there is no gain without pain. That to pursue and indulge pain is desirable otherwise, in this instance, you're not really having the full experience of being a mother.
The gender pain gap goes way back.

Sucking on gas and air

James Young Simpson strongly disagreed. His daily work involved the experience of women in their earliest phase of motherhood. The Scottish-born obstetrician, specialising in the branch of medicine and surgery concerned with childbirth and midwifery, was a renowned and forceful character in the field.

We're taking a step back in time now, to the mid-1800's, to meet Simpson who had always been ahead of the curve. Aged just 14 he started his studies at the University of Edinburgh and was awarded his doctorate at 21. He immediately began lecturing at the same university and, just seven-years later, was made chair of obstetrics. His private medical practice thrived too, with women from across Europe travelling to Edinburgh to be seen by this leading physician. In 1847, at the age of just 36, he was already President of the Royal Medical Society of Edinburgh and had recently been appointed as one of Queen Victoria's physicians in Scotland. He was, however, particularly grateful that he hadn't been called upon during her recent tour of Scotland with Prince Albert. It coincided with an especially busy time and he believed he was onto something big.

Reading this personal attack on his work and professionalism in print, he struggled to articulate a response. Wider tensions had been high for some time between England and Scotland; medical circles were no exception. It came as no surprise to Simpson that his proposals were provoking hostility from practitioners south of the border. Dipping the nib of his quill into the inkwell, he slowly drew it back towards the paper and began to write.

"Almost as often as the human intellect has been thus permitted to obtain a new light, or strike out a new discovery, human prejudices and passions have instantly sprung up to deny its truth, or doubt its utility, and thus its first advances are never welcomed as the approach of a friend to humanity and science, but contested

and battled as if it were the attack of an enemy."[16]

Motivation to deny truth, or doubt the utility of new discoveries, can be found regularly through history. In the 50-years preceding James Young Simpson's predicament it was most notable in the violent destruction of new-fangled devices of technological machinery.

On 9th October 1779, textile workers in Manchester, led by a young dissenter called Ned Ludd, rebelled against the introduction of mechanised looms and knitting frames in their factory. They're said to have smashed up the new apparatus to show the factory owners they could not simply replace their highly skilled craftsmanship with machines. The 'Luddites', as they became known (albeit, a little like Robin Hood, there is no evidence of Ned Ludd's actual existence), would meet up in small groups at night to attack the factory machinery with sledgehammers and axes. In some instances, factory owners would shoot at these protesters, sometimes resulting in firefights. In the early-1800s, the movement swept across the country – starting in Nottinghamshire and spreading to Yorkshire and then onto Lancashire - with weavers burning mills and destroying factory equipment.

Fundamentally, this was about self-preservation; workers fighting to keep their livelihoods and the status quo. They saw their utility being stripped from them. This also occurred against the backdrop of economic struggle from the Napoleonic Wars and Industrial Revolution, both of which impacted negatively on working conditions. They wanted to reinforce their worth in society.

It's arguably human nature to resort to self-preservation when something new threatens your livelihood and this theme is definitely

---

[16] Early opposition to obstetric anaesthesia - FARR - 1980 - Anaesthesia - Wiley Online Library

seen in medicine. Scientific tools used to improve health often face the internal, and very real threat, akin to medical luddism. If a new treatment is seen to replace the need, or skill, of a specialist – or add a new threat to humans - there may be an argument that this is anti-progress.

So, what was Scotsman James Young Simpson doing to cause such anger? Most scientists stand on the shoulders of giants that came before them. In Simpson's case, the beginnings of his foremost discovery can be found in the same year that mythical hero, Ned Ludd, destroyed his first machine from a young man getting high in his living room.

Heating crystals of ammonium nitrate, collecting the gas released in a green oiled-silk bag and then passing it through water vapour to remove impurities, scientist Humphrey Davy eagerly inhaled the resulting haze through a mouthpiece. The effects were superb[17].

"The first inspirations occasioned a slight degree of giddiness", he wrote in his notes. It was followed swiftly by a "fullness of head" and "loss of distinct sensation"; what he surmised to be a highly pleasurable and thrilling feeling. Objects became more dazzling, his hearing more acute. He couldn't remember exactly what happened next but he danced around the laboratory "like a mad man" and knew that his motions had been "various and violent"[18].

What the young chemist, just 20, had discovered while experimenting with crystals was nitrous oxide, also known as 'laughing gas'. So, he quickly invited his friends to visit for a party,

---

[17] The Nitrous Oxide Experiments of Humphry Davy – The Public Domain Review

[18] Humphry Davy; 1800; J. Johnson, St. Paul's Church-Yard, by Biggs and Cottle, Bristol in London

the likes of which they'd never experienced before. They described the 'heavenly inhalations' that made them 'laugh and tingle in every toe and fingertip'. It made them come back night after night for more of the gas that made them 'gloriously happy'[xxxvi].

Essentially, Humphrey Davy and his friends were getting high but the potential of this gas was quickly recognised. Samuel Guthrie (1831) discovered the anaesthetic quality of chloroform; Robert Mortimer Glover (1842) tested this on animals; then Simpson was the first to demonstrate the effects on humans during an experiment with friends in which he confirmed that it could be used to put one to sleep. He started to trial it with mothers during childbirth believing it could "allay the pain of labour". According to scientist, Edward Lund, who visited Simpson in Edinburgh in 1849, "he generally gave it by sprinkling it upon a large sponge cut into the shape of a mask which he placed all over the patient's face. He told me that so little does he fear any ill-consequences from this apparently heroic treatment, that he often performs it at his own house and often even allows the patient to walk home 2 or 3 miles, without danger."[19]

This was the first known use of anaesthetic in surgery.

Simpson's motivation wasn't entirely pain relief. He explained that the longer a labour lasted the greater the risk to patient and child, and pain-relief shortened the process dramatically. "The maternal mortality was fifty-fold greater among the women that were above thirty-six hours ill, than among those who were only two hours in labour: one in every six of the former dying in childbed, and only one out of every three hundred and twenty of the latter[xxxvii]."

Regardless, a swell of negativity was growing against his treatment

---

[19] GB 133 MMM/12/2, Manchester University Archives, Special Collection

with comments and articles warning against the reliance on narcotics in medicine. That the skill of the practitioner should not be surpassed by these uncontrolled substances. Covert meetings would take place at the Crown and Anchor pub in Covent Garden; physicians ranting about the dangerous practice of Simpson, condemning 'ether' as a threat to the patient and their field[xxxviii].

There wasn't only scepticism in quiet corners of London pubs. Oliver Wendell Holmes, one of the most eminent Supreme Court Judges in the United States, said at an address delivered before the Massachusetts Medical Society Annual Meeting, May 30, 1860: "Throw out opium, which the Creator himself seems to prescribe, for we often see the scarlet poppy growing in the cornfields, as if it were foreseen that wherever there is hunger to be fed there must also be pain to be soothed; throw out a few specifics which our art did not discover, and is hardly needed to apply; throw out wine, which is a food, and the vapors which produce the miracle of anaesthesia, and I firmly believe that if the whole materia medica, as now used, could be sunk to the bottom of the sea, it would be all the better for mankind, and all the worse for the fishes[xxxix]."

As we now know, anaesthetic was eventually accepted and heralded. The 'gas and air' offered during pregnancy today is not too dissimilar to that early treatment in Edinburgh. Too quickly, through the centuries, have people labelled new discoveries in science as 'morology'; the study of foolishness, taking the field a step backward rather than forward. Another Edinburgh practitioner put it succinctly at the time by claiming the abuse and vilification Simpson received for his discovery was commonplace and the "reception of almost everything new and great in practical medicine."

Proving a point

In the early embers of his career, Professor Ray Powles had been seen as a morologist. As a foolish pursuer of something nonsensical; someone that, in the sufferance of elongated failure, would surely soon reach his senses and chase a medical field of less folly.

Ray, however, knew the rule. All new and futile scientific pursuits are nonsense until, importantly, they are not.

One person that didn't dismiss Powles' passion for the impossible was Frenchman, Georges Mathé. We met him in an earlier chapter; pioneering bold new treatment with the young scientists of the Vinca nuclear disaster. As Powles ventured into this new specialism of blood cancer in the 1960s, he found himself working under the renowned physician in Paris learning all about the incredible treatment of the victims of the Vinca nuclear disaster. While most wrote-off their pursuits as futile, Mathé and Powles felt they had to find a way to treat some of the most serious blood diseases and the most serious of them all was leukaemia.

As we already know, leukaemia is cancer of the body's blood-forming tissues, including the bone marrow and the lymphatic system. The results are swollen lymph nodes, recurrent nosebleeds, tiredness, frequent infections, weight loss, bleeding, and bone pain. If left unrectified, it will certainly lead to death.

For scientists focusing on leukaemia, the efforts of their peers in the area of immune deficiency – like Jack Hobbs and the team at the Westminster - were a little 'lesser'. Transplants for those people had been happening for some years. The bar was much lower, in their opinion, despite both groups needing to leap through the allogeneic barrier. That is, to introduce tissues or cells that are genetically dissimilar, or from another individual in the same species.

Leukaemia was trickier, like it had a malicious intelligence. A person's own blood cells causing the intricate system to fail. To fully understand those dangerous cells, and tackle them, they needed to observe them at close quarters.

Powles and Mathé had spent five long months counting and separating leukaemia cells thanks to getting their hands on a miraculous piece of kit, called a FACS machine, from the States. More on this incredible device in a few chapters time. There were only four in the whole world, owing to being so new and expensive, but the pair persuaded their institution to invest the $50,000 (something in the region of $500,000 today). Blood entered the machine through a tube, was centrifuged and then dropped into a number of cell collectors dependent on the type of cell they were. Where photographic imaging had previously allowed scientists to inspect around 100 cells every second, this machine allowed them to inspect 20,000.

And yet still, despite all the technical advancements and a much greater ability to inspect leukaemia cells, patients still died with almost 100% certainty. The medical luddite vultures continued to circle.

Returning to London and a role at the Royal Marsden Hospital, working alongside radiologist, Ann Barrett, Ray Powles set about this leukaemia challenge afresh. His cell sorting machine came with him and he soon realised it could be used in different ways. For patients with myeloma, he'd extract the blood and send it for a little spin in the machine. By separating the plasma in the blood that was faulty, he'd exchange with brand new (and functioning) plasma. A world first, but not entirely fixing the overall problem. He kept going.

By the early 1970s, there was renewed global interest in bone marrow transplantation. Since George Mathé's grafted survivors of the nuclear accident in 1958, success rates had plummeted and interest (and investment) in the field waned.

As more patients died and treatments barely scratched the surface.

But there was a new air of the possible. On both sides of the Atlantic science and medicine were starting to see signs of progress. In 1968, Robert Good in Minnesota had performed the first bone marrow transplant on a five-month-old boy with immune deficiency. By all accounts the boy was doing exceptionally well and had a strong prognosis. It bred confidence.

Testing on animals was yielding results too and, with a greater understanding of stem cells thanks to Till and McCulloch in Toronto, a realisation emerged that human tissue typing (HLA) could be the key to unlock the mystery. Ignoring the naysayers, Professor Ray Powles achieved something remarkable in 1973; he was able to successfully transplant the bone marrow of seven-year-old who was living with aplastic anaemia. To achieve this he'd physically intercepted a peer, Rainer Storb from Seattle, who was travelling through London on his way to Germany. We'll meet Storb properly in a few chapters time but this mild-mannered 'kidnapping' enabled Powles to copy a treatment plan which he stuck to religiously. It produced a brilliant outcome.

It was a one-off success at this point but Ray felt he had matched his counterparts, and even surpassed them. He reiterated his view that his specialism of leukaemia was much more complicated. With other blood diseases, there was something lacking (like functioning white blood cells) that needed to be replaced. With leukaemia, on the other hand, something was lurking and thriving below the surface, produced by the body to kill the body. Fixing a deficiency was more straightforward than reversing self-destruction, he argued. Continuing to work closely on trials with Professor Ann Barrett to irradiate the patient's existing stem cells, Powles aimed to totally replace the immature immune system and fix it up with a fully functioning new model. But this was easier said than done and the pair encountered more issues. Radiation was brutal. It blasted every cell in its path, obliterating and subduing until they no longer functioned. There was no way to identify between cells, good or bad, so in attacking the leukaemia cells there was no alternative but to collect some collateral damage. It was delivering as much harm as help. He needed an alternative.

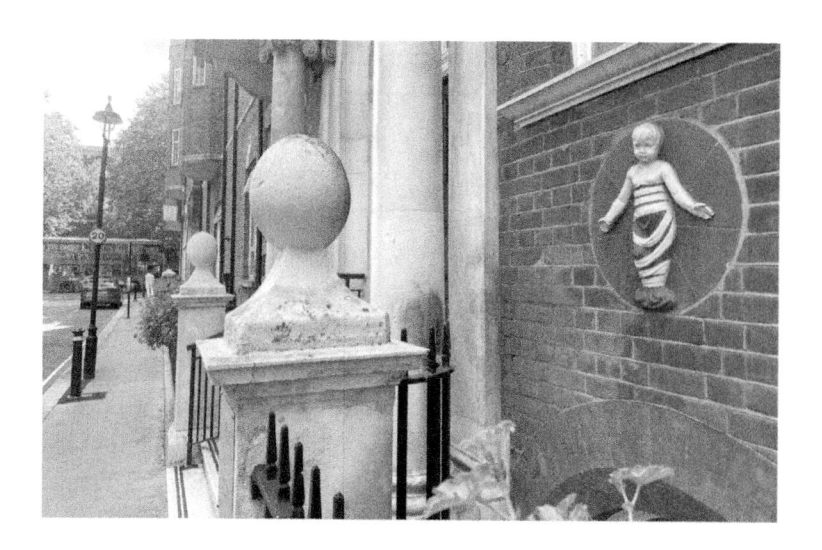

THE TRANSPLANT

13th April 1973

Hunched to the right side of the top step, Liz curled in upon herself for warmth; legs crossed, elbow resting and forearm vertical, cradling a depleted cigarette between fingers an inch from her mouth. Since setting it ablaze the morning light had transformed Udall Street; once smothered by night's dark filter, now awakening with the soft tones and increasing volume of a capital city.

Her last two years had felt washed with muted neutral shades. Now, languishing powerlessly in a shallow darkened despair, she floated face-up, under an immovable layer of a grey film rendering everything as dull, lacking colour, lacking life. Engulfed in Andrew's shadow, she resigned to the stillness of sorrow. As soon as her first child died, she needed to care for her second; stricken with the same disease, destined for the same end. Being here with Simon meant reliving Andrew's pain; each mirrored procedural occurrence, each replicated appointment injured her anew. Nothing appeared positive. The world felt cold, colour dispersing like heat through an open window.

The embers faded; she'd forgotten she was smoking. Her face had involuntarily formed a scowl, the cherubs her focus. Decorative sculptures of children adorned the walls of the hospital, blue and white draped in cloth, identifying this as a place of refuge for sick children. Their faces are resigned. Not pained but ambivalent. Fleeting visitors. The souls of dead children affixed to the exterior as children expire inside. Passengers that travelled fixed pathways in a world they never made. She hates them. Cherubs are tied to religion and, while Liz had a newfound relationship with Christianity, their depictions outside the hospital implied acceptance; that upon leaving here they'll be cared for by a God. That a God can look after her son better in death than she could in life. She heard herself swear out loud, immediately checking around to see if anyone heard. She put her faith in a higher power, and would accept some divine intervention right now but, if that wasn't forthcoming, she'd refuse to be shamed as a bad mother. Not by anyone or any God.

Reflecting on the last few months, Liz knew she'd done all she could to get them to this point. Dragging herself up from the pit of despair, in the wake of unimaginable anguish, she had left no stone unturned in her battle to keep her second child alive. Each decision with the shadow of mortality ever present in the corner of her eye. It pushed her on; while she ignored it, she despised the way it stalked her family. It spurred her to do more, to continue, where some may have stopped. She hated it when people said things like that. 'I could never have done all that you've done', or 'you have a special power to keep going'. What, precisely, did these people see as the alternative? Show her a parent that downed tools when it was in their control to save their child. And now it seemed she could be on the verge of actually saving him.

It was on a walk to St. Albans with her mother, Mollie, just a few weeks after Andrew's death in August, that the campaign began. Instead of flowers or cards in memory of her lost child, Liz decided to request donations for the Bone Marrow Transplantation team at Westminster Children's Hospital. It would buy much needed equipment for the department as their progress in pioneering new alternative treatments was funded through philanthropy rather than Government. Liz stopped by the Post Office in the town to put up a notice in the window asking volunteers to be tested.

The doorbell rang in November and a middle-aged reporter stood flashing his business card, emblazoned with the Evening Echo logo, a local Hertfordshire paper. He'd seen the advertisement while posting some letters that morning and headed straight to the cottage, curious to know more. Liz was surprised the notice was still in the window these months later but, while Simon played inside with Grandma Mollie, Liz sat the journalist down on the outdoor step to explain the dire need for equipment to keep her only remaining son alive. And that time was not on their side.

The odds were stacked against Simon. His rare condition meant there was a one in 50,000 chance of finding a suitable tissue match to make the bone marrow transplant stick. She didn't understand the detail, or use all the correct science terms, but knew plainly that the odds were not favourable. "Then surely, don't you think, the only way to save your little boy is to publicise his urgent need?" Silence hung over across the front porch as the reporter waited for his question to land. It had been a bold move; he wanted to run the story, for sure, but the way he said it affirmed thoughts Liz had already been having. She wouldn't let her son go down without a fighting chance. She felt she'd failed Andrew by acting too late, that wouldn't happen again. She would need the go ahead from doctors at the Westminster, no good would come from antagonising them with unwanted media coverage at this stage. But in the few seconds of pause she had already made her mind up: she'd let them publish regardless. After all, it was only a local paper and it could possibly bring in a few hundred quid to their cause.

On 5th December 1972, the Evening Echo's front page read, 'Hunt to Save Doomed Baby' and the accompanying photo featured Simon sat in a wicker chair, flanked and supported by Liz. Steve Crowther's report led Tuesday's publication and Mollie read aloud the opening paragraph as Liz poured their coffee: 'Simon Bostic will die in a few months unless someone with rare blood can be found to save him". It gave her a jolt and stopped her mid-pour. She'd never heard it said this way before but it was, of course, quite true. Simon played with his toys by the telephone table and Liz, pouring again, motioned to her mother to continue.

That's how it started. The department at the Westminster Children's Hospital had given their consent for the story to run but were hesitant of wider publicity. The procedure they proposed had never been achieved before and too much attention on Simon, a guinea pig with no alternative options, could come back to haunt them if it failed. They needed that improbable close match. That one needle in 50,000 haystack. They had no choice but to support to the cause. It was just the beginning.

A media frenzy began in earnest by February 1973. Simon's face appeared on the pages of national and international newspapers, tabloid and broadsheet, pricking the attention of households, cafes, pubs and commuters across the country – and indeed other parts of the world. His straight, blond hair flopped across his face, his sharp blue-grey eyes coaxing the readers' attention to learn more. You couldn't tell he was sick in these photographs – a happy, smiling young boy juxtaposed with devastating survival prospects written alongside. Headlines such as 'Can You Save this Boy?' and 'Last Hope for Little Simon', all included quotes from Liz and Roger about their fears, about their desperation, about Andrew.

The public response was immediate. The hospital switchboard was jammed. People from across the UK were offering to be tissue type tested to see if their blood fit the bill. Reporters turned up to the cottage in steady succession, all hungry for the latest developments, to discover how close the family were to finding a donor. Strangers arriving at the door brought their own threat to Simon; his immune system so fragile Liz couldn't allow all and sundry to traipse through their home.

She'd position them in the small outside porch, offer them a cup of tea and a comfortable lean against the white, wooden frame as they lapped up a mother's pain. She introduced a plastic garden chair after the first few visitors, easy to wipe down ready for the next. Liz's pedantry was purposeful and necessary. As the weeks progressed each tabloid made it their mission, along with their readers, to save Simon's life. While there were perhaps hundreds of children suffering similar conditions, the Bostic family story gripped a nation, stimulated donors for the bone marrow programme and sold newspapers.

Liz was getting into the role, almost thriving with distraction and renewed purpose. It was surprising, even to herself, how eloquent and knowledgeable she came across, without a hint of nerves or noticeable stutter. When you have a passion, and words originate from the heart, there is no space in the consciousness for anxiety.

She noticed her own skin blemishes in the photos, of course, but perhaps others may not. During 1973, Liz was interviewed on Radio 4 and later television cameras positioned themselves in the back garden, sufficiently distanced from her boy but enough to make her nervous. Their footage showed Simon playing in the sand pit, hugging his mother, making friends with the camera crew and poking the fluffy boom mic. It suitably portrayed the story and pulled the heart strings. She was becoming increasingly savvy to the needs of media. Bleakness still engulfed her days but mostly her nights. Even as spring revealed itself the colours were drained, and so was she.

By now, the search for a donor was on. Blood samples arrived at the Westminster Children's Hospital from potential matched donors everywhere. People making calls to the Children's Hospital were met with 'hello, are you a potential donor for Simon?' and the search had stepped up across Germany, Belgium and Holland. The staff team were inundated but happy for it. Dr David James, burrowed away in the basement broom cupboard, upgraded his shoebox of potential donors to a filing cabinet in the hallway. And soon after a second filing cabinet was needed. In one instance a flight from Washington, DC, brought samples from the United States where Simon's story had made some publications, but the donations had mysteriously disappeared by the time it landed at Heathrow. A newspaper reported 'Mercy Jet Searched for Lost Blood', adding to the heightening drama of the urgent search for her young boy. When the samples were eventually found in an ice container, they proved to be unsuitable matches for Simon.

The problem wasn't with the blood type; Simon was 'O Rhesus positive', one of the most common. It was his HLA, or tissue type, that was much rarer. One Daily Mail journalist called it the search for 'Mr HL-A 1.7/1.8', which was the tissue type Simon needed.

The tone of the media coverage switched in March 1973. It focused on the generosity of strangers and Liz pleaded and expressed gratitude in equal measure. The truth was, they were no closer to saving their son. Even the reluctant doctors had stepped up their involvement in the media, noticing that for the first time ever their small department at the Westminster Children's Hospital was receiving national and international attention for pioneering work. Liz spoke frequently with the team, primarily Professors Hobbs and Humble, who were often asked to clarify the situation in newspaper articles.

Still sat on the step, Liz took a drag of her long-since unlit cigarette. A young couple, perhaps in their early twenties, carried their sleeping child up the hospital steps where Liz sat. She smiled politely as they ascended but, in reality, barely lifted the corners of her mouth. Were they prepared for the ordeal that surely sprawled out before them? Is the attention placed on her son detracting from the treatment of other children in the hospital? She knew that not to be the case; the medical team were incredible, with all the families. But she didn't care if it *was* true; she'd already suffered the loss of a child and shouldn't experience it twice before they had but once. It wasn't a thought she was proud of, her incandescence sometimes got away with her but, she spoke it internally, so who cared?

The door clinked behind her. Would that child find a match? She waded through cloudy memories of an idea in the green room. A vision she'd imagined; a neverendingly long line-up of donors, standing in a corridor, waiting to be called forward. Someone in a lab coat at the front, Dr James, scrolled his rolodex. An archive, of sorts, could match people together. She didn't have time for that now, it would have to wait.

Down the steps and onto the pavement of Udall Steet. As the butt end of her fag tumbled top-to-tail through the air she yanked up her sagging trousers. They used to fit; her clothes now slouched, like her shoulders. She heard it twang the base of the bin. She glanced the way of Vincent Square. Dew coated the grass, a wave of green with white tips like thousands of tiny Christmas trees. The hospital pulled her in. Liz was exhausted by it all. She turned to make her way up the steps.

People die only once. But Liz felt she had died already many times. They would begin preparing Simon for the procedure in the next 10-minutes and she wanted to be there before they started transplanting. Through the entrance atrium, passing big brown doors and dark foreboding hallways. People dressed in white busied around the second and third level balconies, all visible from the concourse. The transplant was scheduled for 8am. Liz ascended the red lino stairway towards the Gomer Berry Ward on the second floor. An energy in her eyes was countered by a lethargy in her step. Despite her earlier blasphemy, Liz was a Christian and believed in God so had no time for superstitious thoughts around the day being Friday 13th. Indeed, it was a Good Friday. She truly hoped so.

The procedure sounded so simple she sometimes wondered why it is so troublesome. They take bone marrow from the donor and put it inside Simon, replacing his faulty cells that don't fight infection. Like moving to a new house, the old tenants take everything with them leaving an empty shell. It may take a few weeks for the place feel your own but then it'll be yours. These new blood stem cells would settle and make a home for themselves inside his bone marrow, producing new, fresh and healthy blood to keep him alive and get him back to full health. It would bring back the boy she knew for his first year of life. If only a donor had arrived in time for Andrew - this trial could have happened last year, perhaps he'd still be here.

She stopped herself; nothing could bring him back. Time to focus on the task at hand. Ward floors were being noisily polished, a large machine with circular buffers swinging freely and uncontrollably from side to side at the hands of the distracted porter. Pale pink paint flaked off walls and radiators everywhere.

She turned the corner to Simon's room; the junior doctors were doing the final checks in their theatre scrubs, masks and gloves in his cubicle. He didn't see her looking through the glass but appeared content with his 'special friends', as he called them. It gave Liz great relief that he'd become so fond of the medical staff at the hospital. He trusted them and it calmed him. She wished for some of that blind faith.

This whole thing very nearly didn't happen.

For months the Registrar, Dr Hugh-Jones, had emphasised the importance of Simon remaining free from infection before, during and after any operation. A matter of life and death, he repeatedly stated; that anyone going into his cubicle could take in miniscule germs that poor Simon would not be able to fight off. Yet there was no 'keep out' warning on his cubicle door, his food came from the general kitchen and nurses kept their gowns inside the cubicle meaning, if only for a moment, they'd need to walk in with unsterilised garments in order to change.

Liz had been furious. What other risks have they ignored? She'd done everything possible to protect him but these oversights could kill her boy. And where the hell was his protective bubble; the sterile tent erected around the bed to guarantee no germs could pass to him? She immediately stormed down the hall to the Sister's office, where Dr John Barrett was scribbling away at his notes. Liz demanded to see the consent forms. They'd been asking her and Roger to sign them for the last few days, unsure when the transplant may take place but hoping it may be soon. She grabbed it from the nurse and instantly ripped it into pieces, astonishing a small gathering of the bone marrow transplant team and a few onlooking parents. As fragments fluttered to the ground, she told them, "I am not satisfied with the precautions being taken against infection and he's not having the transplant until I am."

Dr Barrett explained that there were only two sterile tents, or bubbles, in England at that time and staff needed six-weeks training to know how to properly use them. This riled Liz further. With the consent form strewn across the linoleum floor, she turned on her heels assuring the transplant team she wouldn't be taking any risks. The entire procedure, should there be a donor, was cancelled. Her back to the onlookers she strode down the corridor, terrified but excited by what she'd just done. No time for regret; this would force some changes.

From one exhausting argument to the next. When Roger found that Liz had cancelled the transplant he was enraged. She'd cancelled a procedure that could save their son's life. She'd brushed him aside. "As things are it might kill him", was her unrepentant retort. All this was just a few hours earlier and, until she received the call at the pub, the whole thing was off. Months of media coverage, thousands of pounds contributed from the public and donors across the world stepping up to save her son with their blood, all dashed by ripping up a few sheets of paper.

Liz felt vindicated afterwards when the hospital team conceded that cleanliness standards must be improved on the ward. She let them know she'd be keeping a keen eye on their progress.

Even though the consent forms had been unsigned, and in the bin, the transplant team went ahead and prepared the matched donor anyway. Apparently, it was a woman, roughly Liz's age, who was already somewhere nearby. Later the previous night, Liz had signed a newly printed consent form and, while not showing it, was thankful they had not stalled on account of her. She scribbled on a scrap of paper, "Nobody to enter this cubicle unless previously swabbed" and stuck it to the entrance of Simon's room.

As Simon was being readied for the procedure, Liz steadied herself. She took a second to recognise that at this same moment, there was a woman somewhere nearby unseen, completely unrelated to her family, putting her life on the line to save her son. Anaesthesia, not much refined from James Young Simpson's first iterations, used to ease the donor's discomfort during stem cell extraction. A stranger, possibly with her own husband and family and friends, risking her own health to keep Simon alive. What a woman. That a British newspaper had offered to pay for the life insurance on any suitable donor suitable who went ahead with the procedure, merely added to the sense of danger. Who was she? She must be an angel. Such an unknown procedure with unknown outcomes. Nowhere in the world had this hard graft been successful before. She believed in the scientists and their convictions, but could it really be done?

Unlike children with leukaemia, Simon didn't need radiotherapy to suppress his immune system as it was already non-functioning. His was an old-style Victorian cubicle with a sterile smell, white and blue walls, and dirty curtain rails. Simon would notice the other children come and then go; and by 'go', it almost certainly meant forever. Liz realised not much was said between them; he would just wave at the new person taking their place. When it happened curtains would be pulled shut, silence would fall on the ward, no one would say a word. No words were necessary. Her boy had appeared tired after a disrupted night of bloods being taken but was none the wiser about what lay ahead. By this time tomorrow they would start counting the days, each day's blood results indicating the outcome of the transplant. The last remaining option for her son.

She caught her reflection; dark bags drooped from her eyes like bruises, sleep a privilege of the unburdened. She'd beaten herself up so badly she worried there was damn near nothing left to love.

It would take around a week for the doctors to know if the bone marrow had been accepted by Simon's body; that meant the Easter weekend would ironically be spent second-guessing if her son would rise again.

Perfecting the art
1976

Instantaneously, David realised he was screwed. He leaned forward to look left down the aisle where each and every seat was occupied. He'd chosen the back row intentionally. Running a little late he'd swooped through a melee of people outside, seen a completely free line of seats and slid his way along them to the very corner position. Totally out of the way, his lacklustre timekeeping was now masked as the perfect crime.

He wasn't, though, the last person into the auditorium. One by one, as David idly leafed through the programme of morning speakers, his peers shuffled along after him effectively trapping him in the corner. He was pleased to have found a spot at the rear of Lecture Room 1; it seemed this was a very popular meeting but he was now well and truly stuck. As the first speaker stepped up to the lectern, the penny dropped. He'd walked into the wrong room and now, resigned to his fate, was trapped by a ten-strong row of European experts. He would now need to sit through two-hours about the entirely wrong subjects. His embarrassment was his alone, a private trial.

This segment of the 1976 conference, reserved for the presentation of 'free papers', was taking place simultaneously across two venues and he, absentmindedly, had turned up to the wrong one. In strict time slots of 15-minutes, David White would now be forced to endure presentations he'd previously had no mind to hear; a talk by Italian colleagues on insulin-dependency of cell-mediated immunity, another by a Dutch professor all about the spontaneous release of a receptor cell.

David rued his misplaced turn. The fourth morning speaker stepped forward to introduce himself at the lectern, twisting the slide and focusing the lens of the overhead projector as he spoke. David observed in passive submission as the black and white blurs concentrated ever tighter to form the words 'Suppressive effects of the new antilymphocyte agent cyclosporin A'. A furrowed brow formed; what the hell is 'cyclosporin'?

David White had thus far been enjoying the British Society for Immunology's latest spring meeting in London, the second gathering he'd been able to attend. It was mostly a fact-finding mission; a researcher at Cambridge University, he'd been sent by his boss to network and gather interesting research updates from colleagues attending from far and wide.

Since they were launched 20-years previously, in 1956, these gatherings had been held twice a year and served as an opportunity to bring the leading immunologists of Europe and North America together under one roof to share their promising research paths, build collaborative partnerships and, frankly, to let off some steam among like-minded people. It was a place for the gloaters to gloat, the inquisitive to inquire and the immunology world to picks faults, or heap praise, on their peers. The guestlist was a who's-who of immunology and transplantation from the leading institutions across the world.

Cramped in the corner of the lecture hall, David accepted he had no alternative but to try and make the most of his accident. The Swiss researcher opened by explaining the story of a soil sample he grabbed while on a family holiday in the beautiful Hardangervidda region of Norway. He was a somewhat reluctant presenter, speaking softly but with pace, his English flavoured with a Swiss-French accent. Pretty soon, David White could feel himself leaning forward in his seat; his hands fidgeting, his brow furrowed. This time, not searching for an escape, but desperate to understand more about what chemicals lie within these clumps of dirt.

The speaker was Zurich-born scientist, Jean-Francois Burel. He worked for a Swiss laboratory in Basel called Sandoz, of which David was vaguely familiar, and they were currently focused on testing bacteria and fungi that might be used to make chemicals. Originally, they sought an alternative to penicillin with the hopes of making a lot of money. The more Burel spoke, the more White began to really listen.

Jean-Francois Burel was adamant that, while the research was in its early stages, this new agent he'd named 'cyclosporin' could knock out the T-cells in rats. It meant, he asserted, the immune system didn't fight against a new organ transplant. Just another immunosuppressing drug, White thought. But what was particularly interesting was that Burel claimed this drug would *only* target the immune system, having little to no impact on any other cells.

Burel explained, "what we have found is that in contrast to other immunosuppressive agents and to cytostatic drugs, the weak side effects on the blood stem cell tissues suggests that its action may be directed mainly towards the immunocompetent lymphocytes.[xl]"

White immediately recognised the potential. Back at the Department of Surgery in Cambridge, he and his boss, Roy Calne, had been conducting trial after trial of organ transplants on rats, dogs and pigs but any immunosuppressing drugs they'd introduce would also unintentionally damage, or knock out, other important cells. Red blood cells or platelets would also be killed, stopping oxygen travelling around the body or overturning the animal's ability to clot. If what this scientist was saying was true – that this new agent could exclusively subdue the immune system - it could transform the success rate of organ transplants in animals and, as a result, one day in humans.

It is worth noting that animal testing was then, as it is now, incredibly prevalent in clinical trials. Before testing new drugs or procedures on humans, consensus in the scientific world prevails that you must get it right on animals first. Including this detail, some of it a little graphic, is neither an endorsement nor challenge to this practice, simply a factual depiction of how medical knowledge has progressed over the years.

Back in Cambridge, the number of dogs dying of failed organ transplantation in the research unit was at an all-time high. The canines would already need urgent intervention, so the scientists had nothing to lose. It was little comfort to owners who walked them in but rarely walked them back out. If this new drug, harvested from a handful of soil gathered on a Norwegian plateau, could stop rejection of new organs, this could be transformational.

As the aisle-trappers filtered out for the coffee break, and auditorium lights raised, David White was desperate to get out. Instead of heading to the exit, relieved his ordeal was finally over, he made a direct play for the front of the room and for one of the speakers. Burel was sorting his papers as he sat alongside his Swiss colleague Hartmann Stähelin when, without hesitation, David approached to introduce himself. *"I'd like to discuss getting a sample of this 'cyclosporin' drug for transplantation trials at Cambridge University."* It didn't take long for the Swiss to agree to sharing; name-dropping David's distinguished department lead, Roy Calne, saw to that. It would be sent immediately upon Burel and Stähelin's return to

Basel.

Dog days

True to their word, a few weeks later the sample arrived at the Department for Surgery in Cambridge and the team got straight to work. Calne and White led the initial experiments on the dogs currently in their care and, very soon, they realised this was a drug of immense potential. The minor problem they were finding, with the cyclosporin, was that it could only be administer orally. They'd tried to inject the drug into the dogs but it didn't dissolve in water so was unsuccessful. They figured that it could be successfully dissolved in alcohol[20] but the risk of intoxicating a pack of rather large dogs was a step too far for the scientists. A lab assistant, originally from Greece, decided to try dissolving the drug in olive oil. Who knows why he had the idea but, after visiting a local Greek deli and picking up a specific type of oil he recognised from home, he started to administer the cyclosporin to the dogs with olive oil. It seemed to be working.

Pretty soon the shed at the bottom of Roy Calne's garden was full of dogs. Poodles, Alsatians, Golden Retrievers; normally larger dogs, all of them surviving the rigours of organ transplantation to the point that there was no longer space at the laboratory to house and observe their recovery.

The dogs just wouldn't die. They were living so much longer post-transplant, and taking up more space, that the staff team needed to take it in turns to accommodate them at their own homes. A

---

[20] As part of the initial tests, Burel had administered the drug to himself but had needed to drink two bottles of wine in order to get enough cyclosporine into his system. His colleagues had a struggle managing the trial after that.

problem, especially for David who didn't really have the space at his house for a big dog (or three), but a very exciting problem. Cyclosporin, administered to stop their white blood cells initially rejecting the new organ, was a triumph. The dogs were accepting their new livers and kidneys better than ever before. The Cambridge team knew, beyond doubt, that this drug could potentially transform human survival of organ transplantation. Roy Calne stated that this new drug was "sufficiently non-toxic and powerful as an immunosuppressant to make it an attractive candidate for clinical investigation in patients receiving organ grafts." He'd continue testing it on dogs and pigs and write up his findings in The Lancet; there wasn't enough evidence yet for human trials.

Research lecturer, Raul Scott Pereira, had been keeping a keen eye on the progress of his colleagues Calne, White and co. An immunologist himself, he delighted in his hybrid role conducting research and delivering lectures between the urban Westminster Hospital and the rural University hospitals of Cambridge, primarily, due to his quirky lifestyle choice of waterway travels living on a canal boat.

Pereira, originally from Rio de Janeiro in Brazil, chose the British waterways as his place of residence with his wife and children. The freedom he enjoyed bobbing on free-flowing bodies of liquid juxtaposed starkly with the rigid and structured study of free-flowing blood through the microscope. He'd selected this career after the death of his sister at a tragically young age back in Brazil. She'd had leukaemia as a child which had ended her life and, from that moment, Pereira was determined to dedicate his career getting to the bottom of this certain death sentence for children.

Scott Pereira was well connected and respected at the London hospitals he worked at, was asked to deliver a talk to experts about immunology progress being made in Cambridge. He too had attended the Spring conference, alongside David White, and there were many global updates his team at the Westminster Hospital in London would benefit from knowing. In particular, to Pereira, was the progress of the Cambridge team in the use of cyclosporin. He knew the bone marrow transplantation team very well, working closely with them throughout the 1970s, and while this 'miracle' drug was supressing the immune system to welcome new organs, he wondered if it would work the other way around to accept a new host.

Pereira talked with excitement. You'd never envisage he was born in South America; his accent perfectly English, slightly upper-class, a result of years in private education and scientific circles, one would assume. He delivered a succinct yet energetic update of the key takeaways from the conference, leading with the headline of cyclosporin and suggested they got their hands on some to test on animals. No sooner had he stepped away from the lectern was he approached by a figure he'd desperately hoped to avoid.

"We've got to give it a try."

Hobbs' eyes were alive with excited energy. He'd listened carefully to Pereira's explanation of the new drug, this merciless attacker of T-cells and preserver of others, and realised this could be the thing that saved children's lives. Pereira knew Jack was pioneering, and somewhat of a renegade, but that he had an underlying passion to preserve life. Children like Pereira's late sister. Jack also had a desire for his own acclaim. Not so much to see his name in lights, but to have his name authoring world firsts in transplantation, sometimes whatever the risks. OK, perhaps his name in lights.

Pereira had seen this coming.

"No, Jack. This drug is not ready for use with patients. We haven't done enough animal testing, yet. It needs more time before it can go into circulation. I'm sorry."

Jack Hobbs persisted. He was a bombast. In fact, downright

argumentative. Scott Pereira's position remained fixed.

"You're a radical, Jack. We know your ideas and trials are at the cutting edge, but it would be incredibly bad for business if this goes wrong. We absolutely require more time for testing but things are looking extremely promising. We can't jeopardise that. We won't send you samples just yet. To be truthful, we don't trust you would stick to the rules. Plus, there's no way for a human to ingest the drug yet as it only dissolves in olive oil."

Pereira returned to Cambridge quietly pleased with the way he'd pacified such a domineering character. Jack had become increasingly frustrated the more his Brazilian counterpart had declined his advances, angrily accusing him of obstruction and sacrificing lives. It was all very harsh, very combative, but Pereira just knew that's how Jack operated. His Cambridge team had discussed this likelihood before he'd even left for London. Jack would insist on getting a sample of this miracle drug but under no circumstances would they allow it. At the same time, Roy Calne was pleading with the laboratory in Switzerland, Sandoz, to invest in this new drug. Burel and his colleagues had seen the potential impact but it wasn't yet deemed financially lucrative enough to pursue much further. The development had stalled. Calne, a global name in this area, became an ally of the drug, and of Burel, and took it upon himself to plead with Sandoz senior management to give this a try. This had to be the priority, not farming it out to others to tinker with treatments themselves.

When Pereira walked into the Cambridge Department of Surgery the next day, Jack Hobbs had already been in touch. He'd ranted about their self-enforced protectionism around the drug, raved about their unwillingness to share potentially lifesaving trials and protested vociferously at their personal distrust, vocalised by Pereira, in his professional capacity to adhere to guidelines they set out. The team felt like they had no option if they were to retain amicable relations.

"On one condition, Hobbs. If we send you a sample it cannot be used on patients yet. We simply do not have the evidence, it's far too dangerous."

Jack agreed.

Within one week of receiving the new cyclosporin drug at the Westminster Children's Hospital, a child patient cringed disgustedly as she swallowed a levelled spoonful of olive oil with a mysterious drug treatment dissolved within.

The morologist strikes again

When Roy Calne and David White turned to their article on page 1323 of The Lancet, on 30th December 1978, they realised that Jack Hobbs was not the only person to pip them to the post.

A strange rumour had been circulating for a few weeks in their social circles about a chance meeting on a plane in Italy that had led to this mysterious new drug, cyclosporin, being used with acute leukaemia patients in London. As Calne's Lancet article came to an end four-pages later, it concluded that "further careful study of this potentially valuable drug will be required before it can be recommended in clinical practice." The very next article also featured cyclosporin. It documented its clinical use in five acute leukaemia patients that had developed graft-vs-host disease, stating that four of these died from liver damage.

It had been carried out and written by Ray Powles, Physician-in-Charge at the Royal Marsden Hospital in London. We met him a few chapters ago, a student of George Mathé in Paris working on treatment for leukaemia patients. Powles was the person that had been on a tiny jet plane between Rome and the small University town that he was lecturing at. A fellow physician shared details of this potentially miraculous new immunosuppressive drug. His first clinical trial on the five patients showed evidence that the drug had reduced the skin reddening and soreness within two days, among all patients, but wrote that more needed to be done to understand dosage and treatment, or 'prophylaxis', of GvHD.

But crucially, of the five acute leukaemia patients, one survived. Roy Calne, who'd carefully and meticulously, spent time testing on dogs was furious. He refused to acknowledge this brazen, and in his opinion reckless, trial on humans. He also hated that he'd been pipped to the post. Professor Ray Powles documented the first treatment of a human patient using the cyclosporin drug and, saving the life of an infant boy facing almost certain death, published the article, blowing all others out of the water. The Marsden, and Professor Powles, were ahead of the curve.

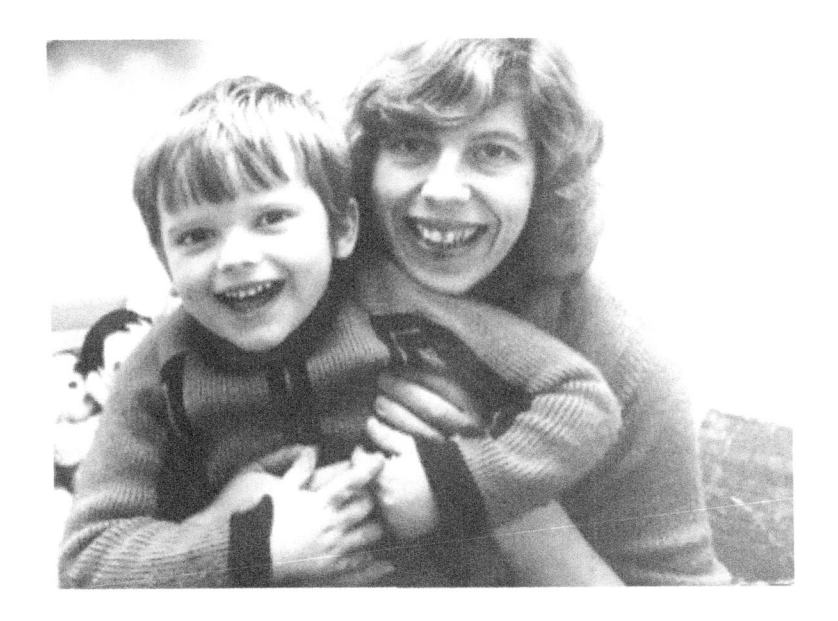

A world-first, perhaps
April-August 1973

Opening his eyes, it took a few seconds for the blurred vision to clear as his body powered-up. Looking around at the whiteness he felt his breath quicken. He saw no one just the emptiness of distant walls encased by the suffocating plastic sheets entrapping him. Blinking water-filled eyes added to his anxiety. His head rested sunken in raised pillows, elevated to see his legs laid out before him. He didn't murmur. He recognised the bed he was in; cold metal bars keeping him from falling, sheets showed Tom chasing Jerry, his favourite cartoon. His breath began to regulate.

Waking from such a deep sleep had unnerved Simon but, all the while, it felt the most natural sleep he had ever enjoyed. Shuffling around he became increasingly aware of himself and took a moment to acknowledge the bandages and soreness he felt around his body. He remembered the tubes, the liquid sent through the pipes into his arm, the cartoons he'd been allowed to watch on the television on wheels. As he stretched his arms and yawned, noticing new pains, he remembered the overwhelming tiredness he'd felt after sitting for hours. Then he recalled no more.

He lay alone. Two nurse outfits hung side by side from pegs, scuffed shoes positioned directly below; a couple of imaginary carers facing away from him, slouched and invisible but for their uniform. The familiar wooden cubicle cocooned him, continuing to curtail his freedom. Dark curtains were closed ahead, almost entirely shut but floating pixie dust caught a glimmer at the edges and he could tell the sun still shone beyond. The last few weeks had gone on forever. 20-month-old Simon knew very little about what exactly was happening to him but what he lacked in concrete understanding he made up for in observed mood. His parents were tense, especially his mum. He'd felt her intense focus on him.

Liz sat crossed-legged in his office down the corridor, left-over-right, her lips pursed. She bade ceaselessly for answers but quietly basked when they were offered. The next few weeks would be key. Since hearing there was a potential success story for Simon, Liz had remained calm. Her diary entry on 15th March read, "Donor found for Simon: washed hair, sunny & warm." They took nothing for granted. Roger eased Liz's hand into his own with no resistance, stopping it twitching from on her thigh. The waiting game continued. They'd keep on as they had throughout, hand-in-hand.

A month after identifying the donor, on Friday 13th April, that the six-hour transplant procedure had been carried out. Then they'd waited. How would those new stem cells settle in their new environment? Liz didn't wish this suspended dread on her worst enemy. She could look at her boy, see him strengthening, smiling and playing like so many others she'd seen on the Gomer Berry Ward before him. But she couldn't see what mattered. She longed to know how the new cells were adapting to their environment. Would they serve as Simon's saviour or plot his demise?

"We've transplanted the stem cells into Simon's system', Dr Hugh-Jones explained. 'We don't know how successful it has been yet, but time will tell. It's a bit like Waiting for Godot. We're confident this is an historic moment – we just can't jump to conclusions."

Hobbs jumped in, with typical confidence. "If one in every ten planes that takes off is guaranteed to crash, it's likely that no one would ever fly. The odds are too risky. But if nine in every ten people that remain on land are guaranteed to be wiped out by war or famine, suddenly those odds of flying look a little less bleak."

He offered stark and insensitive illuminations to merit the decision. He loved to do that, Liz discovered. But she valued his candour. An orator and showman; she imagined he enjoyed the theatre of it all. Simon's paediatrician, Ken Hugh-Jones, continued, "we successfully replaced 12% of Simon's bone marrow with healthy stem cells. That's what we needed. Obviously the more the better but for a child of Simon's stature that should get to work straight away."

That didn't seem like much, to Liz. She sensed that 'HJ' wasn't being entirely honest but, still savouring the thrill of progress, chose not to challenge it. To replace only 12% of her son's faulty bone marrow seemed not worth all the fuss. Will the remaining 88% reject the donor cells? Perhaps adult stem cells, from the donor, were more powerful than her boy's, so the quantity mattered less than you'd immediately think. Either way, the medics seemed energised by the procedure and quickly moved the conversation on to when the family could all return home.

When she walked into the same office a few weeks later, Jack Hobbs was uncharacteristically smiling. Actually, fully smiling. "I've got some really good news for you", he said. "The donor's blood cells have now been confirmed to be in Simon's blood stream. This means that there can be no doubt at all that the bone marrow graft has taken."

Liz couldn't speak. Roger jumped up, elated. He moved to shake the hands of Professor Hobbs and Dr David James, proclaiming relief and gratitude.

Still Liz said nothing.

"Aren't you pleased, Liz?', Roger asked. 'Say something. What are you feeling?"

She was stunned. Unbelievably thankful, after everything they'd endured, but feeling it was almost unbelievable. Could that be it? It was too good to be true.

That same afternoon Simon walked back through the front door of his home at 21 Holloways Lane. For all intents and purposes, that was that. A boy saved; his life could now begin. But it would be a very different experience to when he left. Slowly but surely, he regained strength and playfulness but his house was undergoing a transformation. The fun was drained, replaced by sterile order. Cleanliness was certainly next to Godliness following the transplant; every utensil, every surface, each nook and cranny would find itself doused to within an inch of its life until bacteria was no more. Such chemical purity meant no microbe or cell could survive. Simon was finding it difficult to survive himself. He was a young boy; he wanted to play and get dirty, he wanted to throw toys around and play-fight with his parents. All that was snuffed out by Liz; she felt Simon needed an absolutely controlled environment, like she had fought for at the hospital. Imagine if she'd kicked up such a commotion before his transplant, threatened to call the whole thing off for specs of dust and some cobwebs, only for him to return home and her own level of hygiene cause him to fall ill again. She just wouldn't have it. Every corner of every room of the house was beyond spotless.

As the weeks progressed, and Simon felt more and more himself, he found the situation increasingly stifling. He was made to feel like the feeblest child in the world. His childhood remained hamstrung, maternal projections that he would crumble to dust at the slightest touch. The story of his transplant was now making frontpage headlines, after they'd given it enough time to observe any side effects. There were even discussions of him returning to school in September. Simon was thrilled by the prospect. But Liz's obsession with a sterile home had cranked into overdrive. Photographers and journalists turned up to check on the young boy's progress and Simon revelled in the attention.

He was the first person in history to successfully engraft the bone marrow of a stranger.

Such a wonderful human-interest story. The papers, and public, lapped it up. A monumental showing of what could be possible; of a methodology that could transform the lives of people with immunodeficiencies. But to Simon, he simply enjoyed having his photo taken and getting extra sweets.

Soon enough a media opportunity was organised for Liz, Simon and Roger to meet face-to-face with the stranger that saved his life. Her name was Joan MacFarlane; a quiet and introverted Irish woman, just 28, who'd come forward to help as soon as she realised she was a match. She had a daughter a similar age to Simon and couldn't understand why everyone was making such a fuss about her actions. Anyone would do it, she'd say, if there was a chance to save a life.

Not long after giving birth she'd seen the newspaper articles about this desperate situation; a mother searching in vain for someone's blood to save her last remaining child. Immediately Joan, and husband Bill, went to be tested and were told of the many thousands who had put themselves forward, she was a near-perfect match. She eagerly agreed to the procedure; what other possible option was there? Joan was less than enthusiastic about the media spectacle that engulfed the Bostic family. A photographer busily snapped the encounter, a journalist excitedly asked questions and scribbled notes. The newspaper headline read "Now Simon has two mothers; both of them have given him life", alongside a photo of Joan holding baby Simon.

Back at home, Simon wasn't the only person in the house feeling the pressure. Liz refused to let Roger go to work. He could pick up all sorts of germs and bring that disease back into the home. Simon may not survive it. He was being selfish, he had to put Simon first. But how would they pay the bills? They couldn't possibly stay locked in the home forever. What life was that? They would argue, Simon would listen, continuing to feel somehow responsible for the pressure and stresses inflicted on his parents. Mollie would call almost every day and had a rigorous procedure to go through before she was allowed in the house.

The entry in Liz's diary for 20th September 1973 simply read, "Roger operation, lung removal, St Mary's Hospital". That night she, Mollie and Simon watched the 'Battle of the Sexes' tennis match on TV; Billie Jean-King beating Bobby Riggs. They weren't particularly interested in tennis but it took their minds off Roger's situation. They avoided the hospital as much as they could.

In the home, Simon felt the loss of Andrew through his mother. When she wasn't frantically cleaning, her behaviour was often immovably sad and lifeless. She'd sometimes spend days in bed, one after the next, rising just enough to put food on the table and use the bathroom. You make bargains in grief. An ability to compartmentalise, to turn the tap on and off; to let the exuberant highs of energy follow the slumps of uncontrollable hopelessness. Mollie was around through these times. As if by magic Liz would then jump into life a few days later, cleaning again and feverishly busying herself. She'd do interviews with magazines about her story, take her 'Si' for walks around Brookman's Park and rave about how their lives were back on track. She'd get excited for Christmas, the first they could properly enjoy. As Roger recovered from his operation, and Simon's regular check-ups showed nothing to worry about, Liz's enthusiasm increased.

An unexpected request arrived soon after. Woman magazine, a weekly publication in the UK, wanted to serialise Liz's story. She'd speak with one of their reporters and, over a number of weeks, publish the family's ordeal over the last few years. It felt like the conclusion of a nightmare; the bookend to close of horrid chapter and breath fresh life into what came next. The process felt cathartic to Liz. She'd sit at the kitchen table with a coffee and a cigarette chatting at length on the phone with Rosalie, the journalist. Rules were rules, she would say. It was far too early to risk visitors, especially those from the city.

She'd talk about their dramatic wedding day, her beautiful boy Andrew, the suffering he went through and that maybe he was never meant to live very long. His mission, Liz surmised, was to help doctors learn and save other sufferers. Grieving was selfish; he didn't have any more pain.

She'd call the article, 'For the love of Simon'. In truth, it was a love letter to Andrew and a personal memoir. It had taken incredible determination and a willingness to fight a hierarchy of men in power. The readership loved it.

The media frenzy Liz orchestrated to save her Simon had delivered an unexpected outcome. Not only was she now the world-famous mother of the 'bone marrow boy' but, thanks to her appeals and appearances, Westminster Blood Transfusion Officer, Dr David James, now presided over an exceptionally long, and ever increasing, list of names. They had all turned up to be tested. Their blood type, HLA and contact details logged in the hope they could be a match for Simon. Initially, Dr James added them all to his Rolodex in the basement broom cupboard but he quickly outgrew that. Both the twisting, coloured index and the cramped office-cum-laboratory. Now Simon's donor had been found, and the ground-breaking transplant completed, the list lay dormant. Potential donors not needed, written sequences of phone numbers that would never be called.

Meanwhile, Hobbs was doing his part to write the headlines too. It's unusual for physicians and haematologists to write newspaper articles about their work, normally because no matter how ground-breaking they may be within their circles, the world-firsts are often not of interest to the average reader. Science and medical advancements often get announced sometime later in the globally renowned medical journals, once the submissions have been empirically reviewed and the evidence stacks up to support any claims being made. This is where peers look out for the latest advancements; who is doing what across the world, what has been achieved, what can they learn from things their contemporaries are doing?

In Simon's case, however, Jack Hobbs saw a unique opportunity that he'd long-since determined he would take advantage of. Sick of begging Ministers for money, bored of trying to justify the importance of his department, desperate to see more notoriety of bone marrow transplantation as a lifesaver, perhaps, of many more children. With a receptive British print media, he saw his opportunity to make his case.

Articles appeared in the weeks and months post-transplant quoting Jack Hobbs as he talked about this world first. How he and his team have achieved something previously thought impossible. He reflected on the history; that for decades young children have faced a death sentence if diagnosed with any sort of immune deficiency. But this one boy, and this one team at the Westminster Children's Hospital, have shown it is possible. Now, surely, they will lead the way in teaching others around the globe how to save more lives.

Hobbs enjoyed writing the headlines. He revelled in the glory of it all. And infuriated those around him. Specifically, those colleagues closest to him. Hobbs had worked for years to push the boundaries of what was possible in his field. He allowed others to think bigger, too; not just practically doing things they were trained to do but to challenge if there were better ways to achieve the outcomes they sought. When it came to blood disease, and immunodeficiencies, there had thus far been almost no solutions. They were coming up short every single time. Not just them; others around the world, most notably in Seattle, were failing to make progress either. Pressure mounted on Hobbs. Questions had constantly been asked of the team at the Westminster Children's Hospital. Patients were dying, at a similar to rate to as if the hospital wasn't even standing there, such were the untreatable unknowns. If diagnosis remained a death sentence, why was so much money being spent with no tangible impact.

This line of argument infuriated Jack like no other. He saw himself as the leading pioneer of immunodeficient disease in the world, such was his character, and if anyone anywhere was going to solve this perplexing puzzle it would be he.

With an enthused public audience, and the story of young Simon Bostic captivating a nation, Hobbs didn't wait to publish in the medical journals, he went straight for the tabloid press. He wanted his achievement known; he didn't have time to wait for outside validation to rubber stamp his achievement. He wanted his voice to be the one that told the world.

The papers lapped it up and attention, once again, turned to Hobbs and the bone marrow transplantation team at the Westminster Children's Hospital. The junior team found it invigorating. Doctors Mira Leigh and Caroline Lucas, still overworked and taking their coffee breaks on the wall outside the ward, found it stimulating. Would their whole careers have this energy and buzz around it? They worked insanely long hours together, pretty much living on the job. They'd slump into the staff accommodation on the other side of Vincent Square for a few hours of sleep before it started all over again. They lived on snacks and adrenaline and thrived on it. The camaraderie of colleagues helped ease the emotional toil. Because Simon's success story was still not the norm. Many children died each month, many families still turned to their doctors for guidance, and those doctors still didn't quite know how to deal with that.

Staff continued to taste-check the sterile food; irradiated for safety, staff refusing to feed it to children until they'd experienced it themselves. The children would get so thin it forced the team to question the ethics behind it all. They were doing this to the children, filling them with toxic chemicals and then hoping for the best. Yet spirits were high. Mira and Caroline knew this work was not happening anywhere else and their tireless commitment warranted newspaper coverage. Their families could read the fruits of their labour, their peers could finally understand their field.

It was Hobbs' dynamism that thrust bone marrow transplantation forward; put the field in the spotlight. But the constant risk versus reward, the need for trial and error with human life, caused heated debate among conflicting colleagues that junior doctors, including

Mira and Caroline, witnessed first-hand.

Dr John Barrett believed in dialogue. While treatment, for many, seemed like a no brainer and was little questioned, Barrett never wanted to railroad parents – and sometimes patients - into a decision they didn't quite understand. A transplant came with huge risks; of course, without the transplant the risks were not insignificant either, but he took an approach that was opposed to the typical paternalism of medicine. Rather than the dismissive style of a superior expert informing the lay person how they will get from A to B, Barrett preferred to discuss all available routes and, to the best of his knowledge, any bumps in the road on each path.

When Barrett read the headlines, he couldn't quite believe it. Not only had Hobbs jumped the gun, somewhat, but his 'achievement' – as impressive as it appeared – was perhaps not all it was made out to be.

Barrett was a methodical operator; he played by the rules, meticulously recording data points to choose the optimal course based on evidence. Hobbs was maverick; taking a lead or a hunch and running with it. The pair were never going to see eye-to-eye.

In today's workplace, they'd be encouraged to take personality tests to identify how best to work together. This wasn't so popular in the 1970s and, what's more, their egos would probably refuse to adapt. They loathed each other professionally. On a personal level they would grin and bear it; both had a level of respect for the other and valued that their fundamental motivations were aligned. On the job, however, they were polar opposites; both exploring unchartered territory with the substandard equipment available to them, traversing precarious ice caps with entirely different styles. Neither traversing quietly.

Barrett had an issue with the press coverage. That the young Bostic boy survived, knowing what his family had been through, was obviously a fantastic outcome. But it was very early days. Actively bringing so much attention to this one patient's case could backfire catastrophically. To claim unparalleled success so soon could, if the situation wasn't to turn out well for Simon, cast doubt on the entire enterprise at the Westminster Children's Hospital. To publicly herald a pioneering world first, only for complications to reduce it to yet another failure, could be the final nail in the coffin of bone marrow transplantation.

There was a reason such achievements were published months, or even years, later. Barrett believed it was how good science was done. It afforded them time to be empirically evidenced, for peers to review and replicate, for any unfortunate side effects or outcomes to be observed. He worried that if other physicians copied the process, before knowing the true result, other children may die. It seemed Hobbs was celebrating the transplant loud and proud without the necessary precaution that made it good science.

What's more, Barrett knew everything that was being claimed was not strictly true.

To only replace 12% of the bone marrow with a fresh graft was an immediate red flag. Ideally you would replace 100%, or as close as possible, to ensure the faulty immune system was long gone with no chance to fight back. To only graft 12% meant it was always unlikely the new stem cells would take charge. But Hobbs hadn't explained all that. He'd avoided the caveats and professed his own success.

As the weeks progressed the transplantation team tested Simon's blood and found less and less donor cells in circulation. Ideally, you'd want to see the opposite; Simon's original cells would dwindle and the donor blood would proliferate and thrive. Pretty soon, however, there were basically zero donor cells circulating in Simon's bloodstream. It was no different to the transplants all those years ago after the nuclear accident at Vinca. With no fresh donor blood, to all intents and purposes, the transplant had failed.

Barrett watched as the newspapers continued to monitor Simon's progress; his first day back at school, his mother's three-week multipage feature in Good Housekeeping magazine. He was pleased, more than anything, that somehow this little boy was healthy and living his life again. He sat in meetings where Hobbs championed the ground-breaking achievements of his team, the first group of people to ever achieve such a result. They'd saved the boy from an up-to-now incurable diagnosis – that part was true – but the reason behind that achievement remained elusive. To John Barrett, the science didn't quite add up.

Perhaps young Simon's recovery was thanks to a sudden rush of the donor's white blood cells that immediately set about warding off harmful infections. John thought that maybe the bone marrow graft had helped Simon's body overcome the numerous threats, simply buying some time, to allow his precious few good stem cells to churn out fresh blood. By standing guard and fending-off infections, Simon's own bone marrow was relieved of the day-to-day defence tasks and could focus, short-term, on building itself up again.

In its purest sense, however, the transplant had not worked. That was John Barrett's professional view. It had only been a few months since Simon's transplant and Barrett made it clear to colleagues that the story being portrayed wasn't accurate. It was a false claim; a half-truth. He felt notoriety and commendation was proving more important than precision.

He mused that there may be other motives. Perhaps to secure new funding, gain political clout, put pressure on global peers to up their game. Or simply for Hobbs to gain bragging rights over peers in the United States. Whatever the reason he felt it disingenuous. In the corridors of the children's hospital Barrett's misgivings were becoming increasingly unpopular, especially with Hobbs. It challenged his department's conclusions, called them out them out as false and, while unknown variables meant Simon had survived thus far, Barrett named this 'momentous' transplant a failure.

At a department team meeting in early August 1973, the debate finally erupted. Jack was speaking about trialling the method again, this time with another young patient, when Barrett felt he could remain tight-lipped no longer. He blurted out misgivings, demanded that more understanding was needed and accused his colleague of manipulating the truth to achieve his 'world-first'.

Hobbs' response was explosive. "John, you undermine this entire hospital. The hard work and progress we are making is never good enough for you. Who do you think you are? Respect my expertise. If this unit closes down hundreds of children will die. That will be on you. Do you want that on your conscience?"

Barrett rose abruptly, chair-legs scraping; he turned for the door. He'd never been so insulted. To be scolded in front of the entire department; his professional integrity called into question. Dr Ken Hugh-Jones, a middleman in the centre of it all, tried to calm the situation but others in the room clearly felt the same. A decisive split had formed.

As he reached for the door handle, effectively ending the meeting, Barrett turned directly to Hobbs. *"Blood runs through your veins, Jack, that's where our similarity ends".*

*

While internal debate continued to bubble, Hobbs was still writing headlines. International media picked up on the momentous story and Jack embellished their columns with quotes about the dramatic discovery, his world-leading approach and an end to blood-related deaths; if only investment followed innovation they could move the goalposts for sick children in countries around the world, this news mattered to people everywhere.

Junior doctors, Mira and Caroline, watched John Barrett grab his outdoor coat and storm out onto Udall Street. He probably needed time to decompress. They all did.

Assessing a clipboard full of patient rounds for the morning ahead, the pair found themselves abruptly interrupted as a young woman bound toward the nursing station, emboldened but tired-looking, intent on dialogue. She asked to speak directly with Jack Hobbs and David James – she named them specifically – and told the junior doctors that her son's life depended on it. Her introduction to the Gomer Berry Ward had been nothing short of a whirlwind – a fantastical flurry of noise, frizzy hair and dramatic statements – but her poise and direct demands revealed her to be a woman with clarity of intent.

Asked to take a seat, and reassured that her message would be quickly relayed, she agreed to wait. The specialists would meet with her at their earliest convenience. The woman, just 31-years old, privately welcomed a moment of rest. She was exhausted. Her flight from Australia had only landed a few hours before.

The answers were close-by all along
May 1979

Armand awoke to the barking of dogs. Incessant and repetitive, the snarling in his dream had been significantly more sinister; the beasts that howled and clawed thirsted for blood. Rousing himself, now very much in real-life, he cursed the abrupt wake-up call from the floor below. He must remember to suggest moving the on-call bedroom away from the test subjects. After a quick shower, Armand had a spring in his step. He made his way towards the ward for his shift, exchanging pleasantries with Dr Hickman as their paths crossed on the stairway. Armand chuckled to himself observing Hickman, characteristically fumbling tubes and contraptions, apparatus tucked under his arm and poking out from his pockets. Rounding the corner onto the ward, he customarily wished Dottie a *very good morning*. She smiled and continued scribbling away, perfectly poised she didn't look up from whatever it was she was working on. Affectionately referred to as the 'Dragon Lady', a title she regularly used herself, Dottie oversaw everything in the unit. She ran a tight ship, steering the department with meticulous precision.

Dr. Armand Keating was almost a year into his first medical research fellowship. It was a fantastic opportunity after graduating from the University of Ottawa and the young clinician revelled in being part of such an exciting institute. He especially loved daily clinical rounds on the ward. Since starting at The Hutch, in Seattle, he was always early for these collective tours where specialisms came together; experts in pharmacology, infection, social workers and the transplantation team all walking bed-to-bed together to offer a holistic review of each patient. He knew of nowhere else like it. Such a collective of expertise under one roof filled Keating with a boyish giddiness. He'd discuss hot topics with friends, such as a research trial involving new catheters or ground-breaking advancements in understanding of immunosuppressing globulins, with blank faces all round. But newly qualified, thrust into the most exciting new medical research facility in the country, Armand was in a constant fit of joy.

Something new in Seattle

The goings-on in this facility usually sparked very little public interest. That is, not since the corridors of the Fred Hutchinson Cancer Research Center welcomed distinguished guests and dignitaries for the grand opening ceremony back in 1975.

In the week of their launch, President Gerald Ford[xli] paid a visit, meeting patients in isolation tents and toured the $11-million facility[21]. Other guests including Massachusetts Senator Edward Kennedy, the Seattle Mayor Wesley Uhlman, and Washington Senator, Warren Magnusson who had been instrumental in getting the project off the ground – his wife a patient of Hutchinson during her treatment for cancer. Photographers and journalists were more interested in capturing the sport stars present that day, including

---

[21] President Ford spent approximately 15-minutes at the Fred Hutchinson on Sept 4, 1975, according to diary entries. The following day, when the official ceremony took place, there was an assassination attempt on his life.

New York Yankees Hall-of-Famer, Joe DiMaggio, who had made the trip from the East coast. He was there as this new cancer research institute bore the name of one of the sports most heralded stars.

Fred Hutchinson had been a Major League Baseball (MLB) pitcher for the Detroit Tigers in his playing days and went on to manage a number of top-flight teams until his diagnosis of lung cancer in December 1963. For the next eight-months, Hutch continued to work in his role as manager of the Cincinnati Reds despite undergoing radiotherapy for malignant tumours in his lungs, chest and neck. Given the limited treatment options available at the time the prognosis was not promising for the Seattle-born sportsman but he continued to give his everything for the team until his hospitalisation and death in November 1964. To this day The Hutch Award is given annually to the MLB player that 'best exemplifies the fighting spirit and competitive desire'.

Fred's brother, Bill, was a successful physician who, almost a decade earlier in 1955, had founded the Pacific Northwest Research Foundation (PNRF), a private research institute in his home city of Seattle. The Institute found a home on the site of the Swedish Hospital in the heart of the city, taking up the fifth and sixth floors of Eklind Hall, a former nurse's dormitory. When his younger brother died, with seemingly little science could do at the time to save him, Bill was granted approval from the Board of the existing centre to found a new research institute in his honour, this time focusing on cancer. The foundation stone to the idea was put in place the next year, in 1965, and the plans were bold. It would house 150 staff and support basic research programs in microbiology and immunology, as well as a clinical oncology program with a 20-bed unit. Patients would come here when all other conventional cancer treatment failed. While federal funding was still being secured, Bill quickly recruited his clinical lead to co-found the development of pioneering cancer treatment; a tough Texan called *Edward Donnall Thomas*.

Behind the scenes

Building plans in the works, the medical task at hand was much more complex. A few years earlier, the University of Washington School of Medicine had head-hunted a promising haematology research lead, Dr Donnall Thomas, from the Mary Imogene Bassett Hospital in Cooperstown, N.Y. with a view to creating a leading marrow transplantation unit. Around six-feet tall and balding, Thomas came with an established reputation. Those years in Cooperstown were formative, founding a deep and abiding influence on Dr Thomas' future works.

Back in 1956, '*Don*', as he preferred to be known, performed the first successful syngeneic bone marrow transplant between two humans, a leukaemia patient and his identical twin. To achieve this he'd developed his own brand-new techniques to extract healthy marrow cells and safely transplant them. It was ground-breaking and his seminal paper in the New England Journal of Medicine the following year laid out the future potential of bone marrow transplantation. The problem was that this practice of transplantation was dismissed by leading scientists the world over. They simply refused to accept that the barriers between individuals could be crossed and viability continued to be snubbed for another decade. It wasn't just deemed impossible but, by some, unethical.

A diagnosis of leukaemia at this time was a sentence of death. Why colour in the lines, peers surmised, if you're just painting it black? Almost all cases treated using marrow transplantation from healthy family members later died from infections or severe unpredicted immune reactions. It led to a mass exodus. Physicians left the field in droves, pronouncing it a dead end. Some even called the practice "barbaric", scorning Thomas for actually *killing* patients. Even the recipient of that first twin transplant by Dr Thomas later died when his leukaemia returned. Don's theories countered all the prevailing medical wisdom of the time, and indeed medical outcomes, but the naysayers never managed to deter Don's studies. His rigorous research led him to Washington State to continue this work in 1963. Don's new oncology department operated out of the tired, 12-story U.S. Public Health Service Hospital (USPHS). He hand-picked his own skilled team - some familiar and a few fresh faces - to join him kick-starting the programme on the West coast. He began with his own wife, Dottie; a medical technologist and his long-term research partner. The rest of the team comprised Ted Graham, an animal technician who moved with Thomas from Cooperstown; Dr. Dean Buckner, a medical fellow, also from Cooperstown; Reg Clift, a member of the British Colonial Army who left a medical post in Africa to join Thomas; and Dr. Rainer Storb, a Fulbright fellow who left a position in Paris to move to Seattle.

Trial and error

It is fair to say that the scientists were facing a real battle. Repudiated in medical circles, no one truly believed that bone marrow transplantation would ever work. Despite the indiscreet scepticism, the National Institutes of Health (NIH) did provide basic funding to set up a unit and, for the first four-years, Dr Thomas and the team tested almost exclusively on dogs.

In his prior work over in New York, Don had discovered that dogs could survive lethal irradiation if subsequently transfused with their own marrow. What's more, like humans, dogs adapt to their diverse environments, have a well-mixed gene pool and an ability to develop haematological diseases, including non-Hodgkin lymphoma. Still, it wasn't going to plan. Graft recipients from littermates almost always died due to graft rejection or the common complication of graft vs host disease. By introducing drugs to supress the dog's natural immune system, some of Don's dogs started surviving transplant. It was promising. The canine unit, where Ted Graham would look after the dogs, was down an unused former Navy bunker that had been offered over in West Seattle. It had been left in a bit of a state: chairs flung everywhere, broken tables, office fittings, posters and calendars on the walls and papers strewn everywhere from many years before. But the team used the ample space gladly, taking four-legged patients underground to perform total-body irradiation when they were being readied for transplants. Such was the limited resource afforded to the fledgling department.

By 1969 the team decided it was time to begin transplants on human patients. Don's work had always focused on the possibility of *allogeneic transplants*[xlii]; those concentrating on the replacement of tissues or cells which are genetically dissimilar, and hence ordinarily incompatible, although from individuals of the same species. The decision to begin human transplants was prompted by the discovery of tissue typing in 1968; the success of transplants relied on matching the HLA protein as closely as possible between donor and recipient.

It didn't start well. The first few patients receiving their transplant, primarily suffering with leukaemia, had shown promising signs of recovery following the procedure. The bone marrow of their sibling, or occasionally parent, was settling into its new home nicely and producing fresh blood. Don and the team's theory was that when diseased bone marrow was replaced, the new bone marrow should begin rejecting cancerous cells. But as the weeks progressed the skin began to split, the patient experienced increasingly violent episodes of diarrhoea and vomiting before their internal organs malfunctioned. In a matter of weeks, the patient - often a child - would go from healthy to dead.

Something else that was underestimated in those early days was infection control. The team would do ward rounds and speak with the patients in recovery. More times than they care to recollect they would visit a young patient who was chatty, playful and otherwise looking fine only to listen closer to their lungs and hear a few crackles. A sure sign of CMV, cytomegalovirus, the confirmation that that patient was almost certainly going to die.

Ground was broken for the new centre in First Hill on August 23, 1973. News of the Bostic boy in England sparked excitement. Don Thomas and the team showed this to outsiders as proof in their concept, albeit they were annoyed Jack Hobbs and Co. had beaten them to it. Construction underway, this new Fred Hutchinson Cancer Research Center (FHCRC) institute would stand out as it focused exclusively on bone-marrow transplantation.

Just prior to this, in 1971, the Nixon Administration had announced the nationwide closure of most U.S. Public Health Service hospitals, including that in Seattle where Thomas' transplantation unit was housed. Don would soon head-up the oncology unit when the extravagant new cancer centre opened its doors but, in the meantime, he had to find a way to keep the transplantation work going.

Unlike the Westminster Children's Hospital, the results thus far had been far from convincing but there was, frankly, little alternative. Don negotiated the use of two floors at the Providence Hospital, just the other side of Madison Street, and the team were granted $75,000 to convert the former gynaecology department into a six-bed unit, recruit nurses, a ward clerk, and basically just get started transplanting. It would tie them over.

Our bodies had the answers all along

The pomp and ceremony of the institute's grand opening a few years ago was something Armand Keating had not experienced first-hand, and it was rarely mentioned again. The task at hand being now all-consuming. Approaching the office of lead researcher, Dr. Storb, Armand saw he was still wearing his bright-yellow gilet, running shorts and white baseball cap. Sat at his desk, head-down and not yet changed, he scribbled away at his notes with furrowed brow and face flush. Something big was unfolding, it had been rumbling around for a few weeks.

Rainer Storb customarily cycled to and from the office each day. So acute was his focus on the research, he would sometimes dive straight into the day's work before changing into his shirt and tie. Time on the bike cleared his head. An avid and competitive sportsman, the oncologist revelled in the solitude, passing through and over traffic on the four-and-a-half-mile commute. Of athletic build and standing well over six-feet, Rainer, originally from Essen, Germany, had been part of the furniture alongside Don Thomas since the beginning. In a bold move, he'd written to Don and asked outright if he could transfer across the world to take up a job with him in Seattle. His pluckiness paid off. Then in his late-20s, he saw exciting potential in bone marrow transplantation even if others chose to dismiss it.

Rainer's research focused on one key question: what if the body could naturally fight cancer? If it were possible to manipulate the immune system to attack the cancer cells, while leaving all the healthy cells alone, could you prime the blood to kill cancer?

The foundation of immunology – treating disease and infection through the body's own immune system – is often thought to trace back to Edward Jenner in the 18th century. Smallpox had proved itself a mass killer for centuries and, if you were fortunate enough to fight off the disease, you could be permanently and hideously scarred. While Jenner was certainly not the first to suggest, nor the first to attempt, vaccination of cowpox as a pre-emptive immuniser (the similar method of variolation had been around since the 18th century in India, China and Sudan), his paper led to the adoption of widespread vaccination and prevention of the deadly disease.

Yet when it comes to cancer the power of the immune system remained unknown. In the late 1800s, German physicians W. Busch and Friedrich Fehleisen believed that by injecting a bacteria they could reduce the size of a tumour – a theory later confirmed by the works of American surgeon, William B. Coley in 1909. Around the same time, German physician Paul Ehrlich was picking up the Nobel Prize for his work on immunity. He'd been personally tasked by the German Emperor Wilhelm II to devote all his energy to cancer research, following the death of the Emperor's mother, Princess Victoria (the first child of Queen Victoria of Great Britain), to cancer.

Ehrlich's investigations led him to develop the theory of *Zauberkugel*, or 'the magic bullet'. It seemed somewhat like science-fiction at the time but his belief was that a compound could be made that selectively targeted a disease-causing organism, without harming the body itself. He envisaged firing a 'bullet' into the blood system consisting of a toxin to attack the problem organism, accompanied by a clever agent of selectivity; a sort-of homing-device that would lock-on to only those targeted cells. His first magic bullet, and crowning achievement, was Salvarsan 606: an arsenic derivative that proved effective in curing syphilis and went on to become the most widely prescribed drug in the world.

The foundations had long-since been laid but Rainer Storb knew his latest research paper, published just the day before in the New England Journal of Medicine, had taken it a gigantic step farther. His landmark submission offered unequivocal proof that human immune cells could cure cancer. He argued that by activating our own disease-fighting T-cells in the blood we had a far greater chance of defeating leukaemia in its various forms. That a graft of our own blood could fight the leukaemia.

And the way he testified you could make this happen, bone marrow transplantation.

The phone had been ringing off the hook. Dottie fielded calls from Paris, London, Moscow and Rome – not to mention every cancer centre across the United States. There was a buzz amongst staff, well aware of the theory but energised to see it in print. There was a quiet knowing. Patients and their families went about the ward none the wiser, not avid readers of scientific research journals.

Rainer sat at his desk for most of the morning, unusual for him. He'd typically clocked up around five miles on foot each day, transferring between lab bench and ward rounds, balancing studies under the microscope with observations of patients. He was the steady metronome of the department; the regularity of his patrols reassured those around him. But the more he learned, the more he learned he didn't know. He'd seen too many children die. Too many young lives extinguished in excruciating pain. Too many mothers and fathers broken.

Live or die, transplantation was proving to be a harrowing ordeal. Patients would receive intensive chemo or radiotherapy and the drugs would often make them incredibly sick. Staff on the transplantation team had to administer sedatives to keep them from consistently throwing up. While not totally passed out, it meant they would sleep through the day and night with a view to keep them from dehydration, caused by constant nausea and vomiting. But when they woke, they'd immediately roll over to throw up. Post-chemo or radiotherapy patients found it impossible to eat or drink, the sickness rendering them unintentionally nil by mouth meaning the nutrition levels in their body plummeted making them more susceptible to infection. This would go on for days throughout the treatment and, after the transplant, the medical team would cross their fingers that the patient showed signs of improvement after around one-month.

Rainer's research showed that leukaemia patients who had experienced little to no Graft vs Host Disease (GvHD) had a less than 40 percent chance of staying cancer-free several years after transplant. They were more likely to relapse. Unexpectedly, well over 60 percent of patients who experienced more severe GvHD were cancer-free as many as eight years after transplant. So, while the new blood dangerously attacked the healthy cells, through Graft vs Host Disease, they also attacked and eliminated the cancer cells. Storb wondered if you could manipulate the T cells to attack only the cancer cells then the miracle solution might lay in our blood all along. Unconceivably, a little bit of GvHD would turn out to be a *good* thing. Trials in his newly published paper had shown that, over a 180-day period, almost all T-cells and bone marrow cells were donor – meaning no host cells remained – and the patients were recovering. To uncomplicate the premise, Rainer called it the 'Graft vs Leukaemia Effect'.

Rainer hadn't slept last night. Nor the night before; distracted by whirring self-doubt. Countless condemning voices of cynical peers saturated his psyche, imagined but angrily manifesting in various languages. But his science was sound. He knew the broad implications of this discovery. That GvHD, the very nemesis that callously stole young lives before their very eyes, was the precise antagonist that would become their salvation. Rainer's leg twitched under the work bench, his thumbs toyed in clasped hands, resting on his lap. He was an athlete on the blocks; all the years of dedication and sacrifice had led to this moment, the promise of something spectacular within his grasp. He had fired his own starting pistol. How he hoped he wouldn't regret it.

Weird contraptions

Armand Keating and Robert Hickman passed each other on the stairwell for a second time that morning. The latter was making his way to see Dottie about a paper he was finally ready to submit. Tucked inside a green tabbed folder grasped tightly in his left hand was his latest typed-up offering; his right hand independently wrestled the pipes and cylinders that constituted the crux of his proposal. He knew that Dottie would not want to see a demonstration, the paper must stand alone in its efficacy, but Robert took them regardless, possibly as a source of comfort. Dottie reviewed every research paper produced by the department. Her stamp of approval was paramount to getting it out into the wider world and her mantra was clear; we should *all* be able to revel in the majesty of science. If scientific beauty cannot be enjoyed by an outsider, you haven't done a good enough job of explaining it.

Hickman had been part of the transplantation team at the Fred Hutchinson since day one and the 52-year-old doctor, slightly rounded and long-since balding, was liked by absolutely everyone. Mild mannered, always jovial and seemingly of a perpetually kind disposition to patients and colleagues alike, Robert's devotion to good care was matched only by his dedication to crafting his odd-looking devices. He had a way of looking at people that let them know he was really looking at them and he always smiled with his eyes.

One of the dangerous side-effects of irradiating a person's blood was that it caused patients, mostly children, to lose around 10-15% of their body mass during their treatment. And in the following days and weeks, they would be violently ill, their bodies ejecting the remaining nutrients with no appetite, energy or willingness to replenish them. It was a huge concern for the team. The lower a person's nutrition, and the more weight they lost, the more susceptible they were to infection and the less able their body is to recover from the gruelling treatment for cancer. They'd tried all methods, aside from force-feeding, but even that wasn't off the table as the situation grew unmanageable. They were almost starving to death.

Robert's area of expertise focused on the administration of chemotherapy through tubes, or catheters, into the veins, known as 'intravenous' or IV, as well as all other fluids into the patient's body. Now, you have to remember that the success rate of bone marrow transplantation at this time was incredibly low. The patients you find in these ward beds are in their last chance saloon; it's their one remaining resort.

During the course various treatments over many years their bodies have been buffeted, squeezed, jabbed, scanned, prodded, poked and jolted, both inside and out. As a result, their veins become fragile, used over and over to put fluid in or take samples out. Veins become a little adverse to the attention. Nurses were, and still are, lauded for their ability to locate a usable vein against all the odds. Patients at The Hutch were a particular challenge: as their nutrition and hydration levels plummeted their veins constricted, retreating to the safety inside and carrying less blood around to parts of the body.

A few years ago, back in 1973, Dr Hickman had tried a device on a patient when no other solution could be found. The nurse couldn't locate a usable vein in an advanced leukaemia patient so, despite it never being used on bone marrow transplant patients before, Robert introduced the *Broviac catheter*. Invented by a colleague of Hickman's at the University of Washington, the Broviac catheter passed through a vein in the chest into the right atrium of the heart and allowed for successful delivery of intravenous nutrition. It worked. From that day on, Hickman and the team of Hutch nurses used the catheters to intravenously provide nutrition, the process of alimentation, to patients that otherwise skirted with death during their treatment. But as the years progressed the nurses raised other problems. They didn't just need to put nutrients into the body but take blood out as well, and they therefore wanted a bigger line too with greater capacity.

Hickman had been working on the problem ever since. Every few weeks he'd be seen jovially fumbling around with new tubes and quirky-looking gadgets on his ward rounds, conjured up in cahoots with the centre's engineers. What he needed was a new catheter, an advancement on Broviac's version which kept slipping out, that had additional lumens; the portals through which fluids can pass. He envisioned a single device that could be used to deliver IV nutrition, draw blood *and* deliver chemotherapy. A one-stop shop. This, he believed, could not only transform the experience of bone marrow transplantation treatment but, indeed, all cancer treatment. His prototype was ready.

Steps away from Dottie's door, Hickman froze. Had he missed anything? Would she throw a curve ball? He'd been using his prototype device, in all its iterations, for months now with near impeccable results. But one stone unturned would be unceremoniously excavated by Dottie, strewn to one side and he'd be forced to start again. His new catheter would make the pain and tension of constant punctures and needle sticks a thing of the past for patients.

Dottie opened the green folder bearing the title of his paper on the cover: 'A modified right atrial catheter for access to the venous system in marrow transplant recipients'. If she gave it sign-off and Don agreed to co-author, as he did with all papers from the department, it would reach a global medical audience. As she poured over the pages Robert Hickman expectantly waited, reading into every physical response from her breathing to the way her fingers leafed through the paper. To get this published and release the mechanism to hospitals and paediatric units across the world filled him with an excitement unparalleled. If he could meet the next deadline for the esteemed Surgery, Gynaecology & Obstetrics journal it would be published in the June 1979 edition[xliii]. The *'Hickman Line'*, as it was to be known, would change the game.

The department was experiencing one of the most pivotal months in its history to date. They had their bases loaded; so much innovative research reaching their defining crescendos simultaneously. Pay-checks were based on successful grants, at this time, and no one had a guaranteed salary. Innovation was crucial.

Returning triumphantly from the review meeting with Dottie, tubes and gadgets tucked back under his arm, Robert Hickman framed the lab doorway. "Don's called a meeting in his office. He wants us all there in 10."

Trainee Armand Keating was the last in and closed the door behind him. Simultaneously Don rose from the chair behind his desk and pushed his glasses to rest onto his forehead. His trademark white beard flawlessly groomed, blending as a seamless extension of his pristine lab coat. Softly spoken, Thomas got straight to the point.

"Frances is an identical match for Laura. We'll need to inform the parents, and

get their consent for transplant, but they'd be foolish to say no. This is it."
Stunned into silence, all eyes turned to Frances Otto-Depner. A young clinical lab scientist at The Hutch, she'd often donated her own platelets and blood for treatments but this was different. Against all odds, her HLA type precisely matched a patient on their ward who was in desperate need of a bone marrow transplant. Frances had been consulted and had, in an instant, committed herself to the process. This experimental and unproven procedure posed a huge risk to everyone involved; while Simon Bostic's transplant had taken place in London six-years prior, no American team had never conducted a transplant involving an unrelated donor. This would be a first.

Don pierced the gawping with typical pragmatism. *"So, track down her parents and let's get ourselves prepared."*

Dottie led the team from the office, sideways glances exchanged but no words. Rainer remained behind as Don retook his seat, folding his right-leg over, lowering his spectacles and smoothing the sides of his beard. As the last person left Rainer turned expectantly to Don who, without missing a beat, temperature checked the moment.

"I guess it's time to see if your theory really works."

Caught by surprise
1981

Yellow and blue lights flickered outside bustling bars along the strip as the young couple strolled hand-in-hand down the sidewalk. They'd enjoyed their night. The warm spring breeze kept their skin glistening after a hot but glorious evening of drinking, laughing and dancing with friends at The Living Room café in West Los Angeles. It was sometime around 1am and Santa Monica Boulevard was still as vibrant as ever; traffic flowed and beeped, cyclists straddled pavement and road, some less steadily than others. The store doorways filled with rough sleepers catching a break. The city was alive.

Joel had recently turned 38 years old but he wouldn't hear a word about his 40th. In a new relationship, or at least he hoped this would develop into a relationship, he felt completely reborn. OK, so their first date had been a bit awkward, but he was extremely out of practice. Joel had left his wife five years before, over in New Jersey, and moved across to the West Coast to start afresh. As a young boy his family would always visit his grandmother in L.A. and he loved every minute; mainly the proximity of the city to the beach and mountains, and, of course, the weather. Despite the change in climate, it had taken a bit of time to warm up. A little shy, but slowly finding his feet, Joel started his own business in Sherman Oaks the previous year, 1980, and things were all falling into place. They'd hail a cab and head back to his apartment; it was closer. A Friday night to remember and this new relationship may really be going places.

Back to earth with a bang

Monday morning came around too soon. As Joel turned off Van Nuys Boulevard, into the General Practice parking lot, his business partner, Dr. Gene Rogolsky, drew into his designated spot, a furrowed brow visible through the windshield. Joel immediately snapped back into work-mode; memories of a perfect weekend now banished.

The pair had revelled in the freedom and autonomy that came from business ownership. Both were experienced general practitioners, good and popular ones at that, but over the last six-months an unusual trend had seen them treating new patients from across Los Angeles County and even some from San Fernando Valley. A trend that they couldn't quite get to grips with.

Back in October of 1980, Halloween night to be precise, Dr Joel Weisman has joined a group of friends for dinner. It wasn't exactly appropriate conversation for the dinner table but Joel spoke of patients he'd recently seen that had troubled him, all anonymously of course. They involved unusually high number of intestinal parasite cases and routine illnesses that returned mysteriously, again and again. They couldn't put their finger on it. He figured, he'd told his friends, it was an immune system breakdown, of sorts, and in certain cases a complete failure. Until recently, however, the patients had all been fit and active.

Since that Halloween, perhaps five-months ago, more and more similar cases appeared. It perplexed them both, Gene's early morning scowl evidence of that, and had made the last few months of work both draining and worrisome.

By lunchtime, Dr. Weisman had seen two new patients that troubled him greatly. Both, previously healthy young men, exhibited a disastrous array of confounding problems, including persistent diarrhoea, eczema, fungal infections and extremely low white blood cell counts. But it was strange abnormalities of lymph nodes that made them more anxious. They had no idea what they were dealing with.

Perhaps Gene had had a sixth sense that Monday morning, or one of those unmistakable feelings deep in your gut, because things were about to unravel at unimaginable pace.

A problem shared, is still a problem

Knocking twice on the glass-panelled office door in the basement of the University of California Los Angeles (UCLA) Medical Center, Joel Weisman could feel himself nervous for the first time in a very long while. He felt he'd only seen the tip of the iceberg.

As the door opened, he was enthusiastically greeted by a young immunologist. Joel, still wrestling with nerves, fumbled with papers. This was the man he'd been told he had to meet with.

As more and more patients had turned up to the surgery with swollen lymph nodes and stubborn low-grade fevers, Joel and Gene agreed they could no longer keep guessing and hoping for the best. Something big was happening. Usually, those symptoms would signal the start of lymphoma, but there was no cancer visible anywhere. Even Sylvia Weisman, Joel's mother who worked as receptionist at the surgery, had noticed the common link. It didn't sit well with her, particularly when it could affect her son. Pleasantries exchanged and a coffee in hand, meeting host Dr.

Gottlieb took a steadying breath and promptly sprang into action.

Michael Gottlieb was even newer to Los Angeles than Joel having completed a fellowship at Stanford University in Palo Alto, California just the year before. UCLA itself wasn't completely new to him, though, as he'd spent some time studying bone-marrow transplants there and, as a result, the university invited him to move south and open an immunologic research lab. Clean-shaven, aside from a prominent mousy-brown moustache, he was young, enthusiastic and a little wet behind the ears. With dark curly hair and sporting huge glasses, which covered half his face, he lived and breathed everything 1980s L.A. had to offer. He quickly accepted an assistant professor position focused on the 33-year old's speciality, the immunology of organ transplantation.

Since the turn of the year, Gottlieb and his colleagues had encountered a few patients experiencing the same unexplainable complaints that Weisman had seen in his practice. But their meeting had been arranged for something more specific.

On a slow morning around one week before, in March 1981, Michael Gottleib was supervising the training of junior doctors and the most unusual thing occurred. The young fellow in his charge, Dr. Howard Schanker, was looking to get his teeth into something new and Michael, perhaps out of lethargy or perhaps believing in a medic's intuition, sent the trainee on a patrol of the hospital looking for any patient whose case may present something a little out of the ordinary. A vague quest but a fruitful one. Pretty soon Schanker returned to the basement office with a wide-eyed look of confusion on his face (Fee & Brown, 2006)[xliv].

"There is a guy upstairs whose infections are really kind of strange".

Like Gottlieb, the patient in question was also named Michael and was also 33 years old. He was a tall, good-looking man with short, peroxide hair and prominent cheekbones. He admitted to being a model by profession although, when Gottlieb and Schanker travelled up to see him, they'd never have guessed it. Michael had been suffering with a fever for almost six months and he couldn't seem to shake it. He'd experienced swollen glands in his neck and collarbone but, while those inflammations seemed to have gone down a bit, a new symptom was sporadic hair and weight loss.

It was unusual but the lab tests caught them cold. Michael had raw patches of fluffy white growths; *candidiasis*, a yeast-like fungus, as well as herpes virus inside his mouth, between his buttocks and on his index fingers. The air spaces in Michael's lungs were filled with millions of *Pneumocystis carinii*, a microscopic parasite that attacks cancer patients and recipients of transplants, people whose immune systems have essentially ceased to function. It was so rare that Gottlieb, a specialist in transplant immunology, had never seen a case before.

After observing the tests under the microscope in the basement laboratory, the confused pair had some questions and hiked up to the ward to speak with the patient. Turning the corner into his cubicle they overheard him speaking with a friend on the phone. Quite matter-of-factly, he announced, "the doctors tell me I am one sick queen."

As Gottlieb recalled this account, Joel Weisman's anxiety increased again.

The symptoms his counterpart described were almost the precise indicators he'd seen in his two patients on Monday morning a few weeks ago. The same inflamed lymph glands, the same random hair and weight loss, the same inability to shake a persistent fever no matter how many supplements and resting they committed to. They'd both had herpes, or cytomegalovirus (CMV), in multiple locations and a yeast-like fungus growth. When Gottlieb finished recounting the story, Weisman swooped in immediately to corroborate the findings with evidence of his own.

All three patients were men, each deteriorating in health at a frightening rate and each had attended appointments alone within the last week. Gottlieb arranged to have Weisman's two patients admitted into UCLA for further testing. As they bid each other farewell, both knew this would be the first of many encounters together. Gottlieb shared his perspective with Weisman, that "in medicine, one case of something is a curiosity. Two cases make things very interesting. But a third case, that forces you to ask: Is this going to be something big?"

After the meeting Joel returned to his practice knowing this was taking on a life of its own. Over the coming weeks he would see even more patients with fungal infections and stubborn fevers. This mysterious 'syndrome' was spreading. He constantly challenged the assumption that kept creeping into his mind. Less of an assumption, more of an accumulation of data, but still something he couldn't yet accept. His mother Sylvia had the same concern. Joel considered his own new relationship and how this could impact the two of them. They were still in the honeymoon period, enjoying each moment together, offering such a refreshing break from the stress of the job. This could change everything. If his assumptions were correct, he and Timothy were both at risk.

There couldn't possibly be such a thing as a 'gay disease', could there?

Identifying a killer

On the ward of the UCLA Medical Center, model Michael's outlook continued to inexplicably worsen. Along with the two patients referred by Dr Weisman, there were now a total of five men admitted to the ward with almost identical symptoms. None of them would ever leave that hospital. On 3rd May 1981, Michael died followed shortly after by another of the men.

It was time to sound the alarm. An alarm that would ring out loudly across the entire world.

Gottlieb realised he'd discovered something that could be huge. His tests under the microscope had identified that *CMV* and *Pneumocystis carinii* were present in all cases, that all cases were gay men. Whatever this was had now led to a body lying in the morgue. He wanted to be ahead of the curve. Straight away Gottlieb got on the phone to the editor of the illustrious New England Journal of Medicine. They could splash this headline across their pages, his name underneath as the '*discoverer*'.

"*I've got you possibly a bigger story than Legionnaire's disease*", Gottlieb claimed. But he was told publication would take too long, months in fact. This needed to be out there immediately, so the editor encouraged Gottlieb to write an article to a weekly report journal. This would ensure he was credited but that no time would be wasted informing the public.

Together, Gottlieb and Weisman penned a letter to the '*Morbidity and Mortality Weekly Report*' published by the Centers for Disease Control and Prevention. They outlined their observations, talking of a "potentially transmissible immune deficiency" and suggested it was likely to be sexually transmissible. The pair hypothesized that a new strain of CMV had emerged in the homosexual population and that a high level of exposure to cytomegalovirus-infected secretions may account for the occurrence of this immune deficiency.

For the purpose of labelling, they described it as a 'new acquired cellular immunodeficiency'.

What had been identified by Gottlieb and Weisman in the patients went on to become one of the greatest medical horror stories of the

20th century.

When the editor eventually published Gottlieb's article in the New England Journal of Medicine in December 1981, he went into much greater detail about their findings and how they were able to identify 'GRID', the name officials initially chose for 'gay-related immune deficiency'. This was the disease that would later be known as 'acquired immunodeficiency syndrome', or AIDS.

Gay disease

Our fight against killer blood has thrown up some real curve balls through the years. This one is a monster.

We've momentarily hopped forward a few years here, to the mid-1980s, as gay rights and lifestyle freedoms had reached exciting new levels. For a decade a new generation of young gay and lesbian Americans saw their struggle within a broader movement to dismantle racism, sexism, western imperialism, and traditional limitations regarding drugs and sexuality. Public consensus meant there was no need to shy away anymore or hide their sex lives. But there were still legal limitations dependant on where you lived as a gay individual. For example, the state of Arkansas recriminalised same-sex consensual 'sodomy' with the approval of then-State Attorney General Bill Clinton. In many states, including Arkansas, same-sex sexual activity was illegal up until 2002 – and this was only enforced when the Supreme Court deemed it unconstitutional - no representatives had rectified the statute themselves.

"But that was then and this was San Francisco.[xlv]"

In San Francisco, Los Angeles and New York in particular, Pride Parades and Festivals had grown in size year on year. From their initial iteration as demonstrations in protest to the Stonewall Inn raid in 1969, for a long time in direct conflict with the LA Police

Department (LAPD) who forcefully tried to shut them down, they had become a loud and proud celebration of everything LGBTQ through the streets of Downtown Los Angeles.

For many the lifestyle was colourful, loud and unapologetically sexual.

Finally, people could celebrate their sexuality, promiscuity and true character. As word of the 'gay disease' circulated in social circles of Greenwich Village and West Hollywood, however, the suggestion was often met with distrust in the gay community. A cancer spread by gay sex, they would argue, was just the latest effort of the establishment to subjugate a way of life and new freedoms. After all, where are these so-called GRID victims? There was nothing on the regional or national news channels warning of a health crisis. Just word of mouth, a friend-of-a-friend who'd become sick, no evidence that there was any link to the gay lifestyle. It was clear that self-criticism was not the strong point of a community only beginning to define itself affirmatively after so many years of repression.

People were dying but nobody paid attention because the mass media seemed skittish when covering stories about homosexuals and gay sexuality. So too were many health institutions at the time, not particularly enthused at being known publicly as a hospital specialising in treating gay disease. To be infected was to experience your body under attack. Fit and healthy men would be reduced to shrunken skeletal frames, with painful blotches and breakouts of the skin, difficulty breathing as they drifted in and out of consciousness, totally bereft of energy. Bed-bound, the experience would progressively worsen until death came as a saviour.

Newspapers and television largely avoided discussion of the disease until the death toll was too high to ignore, and the casualties were no longer just the outcasts.

As the months rolled on, Joel Weisman became increasingly vocal about the behaviour he believed was escalating the spread of the acquired immune deficiency. 'Acquired' because the data strongly suggested correlations in the spread. And transmission was increasing exponentially. One of the first cases had been discovered in Denmark, with a health worker returning from Zaïre (now the Democratic Republic of the Congo). When we say 'the first', we of course mean the first 'Western' case because, historically, that tends to be when the world takes notice. After setting up her own hospital in the village of Abumombazi in 1972, Danish physician and surgeon Grethe Rask, became increasingly sick, returning home to Denmark and died in December 1977. The recent spate of diagnoses, however, had until now been fixed to the transport hubs of North America, particularly where there was a thriving gay scene. Weisman's primary concern was the activity in the bathhouses across these transport hubs.

While bathing may have been part of the deal, gay bathhouses, also known as saunas, were a meeting place for men to have sex with other men. They're believed to date back to the 1400s in Florence, Italy, while in centuries since 'the baths' have found popularity in Paris, New York and London. At the North Hollywood Bathhouse, a short distance from Weisman's medical practice, you would slide $13 under the glass panel to gain entry through a door bearing the sign, *"This club caters to adult gay men. If you are offended by any aspect of this lifestyle, do not enter."* Handed a towel as your uniform, attendants would direct you to a fishbowl full of condoms and a shelf of brochures on safe sex while disco music boomed an incessant beat from overhead speakers. This was a legal 24-hour establishment and, if you didn't find anything to your liking, The Corral Club and the Hollywood Spa were just a stone's-throw away, as well as others a little further afield. There was no shortage of choice.

Joel Weisman, an openly gay man operating a medical surgery with predominantly gay patients, was appalled by these places. He saw the bathhouses as horrible breeding grounds for disease. The more he spoke to his patients, and understood their behaviours, the more he saw the links. Certain names kept finding their way into conversations, similarities that went beyond coincidence. People who went to bathhouses were simply more likely to be infected with a disease, and infect others, than a typical homosexual on the street. Weisman, now becoming a prominent voice on this new disease, spoke passionately of how he saw this spreading and steps to take to stop it. Namely, to stop having sex. He was met with mixed responses, from *'they're trying to stop our way of life, our newfound freedoms'* to *'this is an epidemic, stupid.'*

As Randy Shilts put it in his book, *And the band played on*, "without the media to fulfil its role as public guardian, everyone else was left to deal—and not deal—with AIDS as they saw fit"[22].

Hiding in the blood

Imagine you're walking in a woodland area, trees and wildlife all around you, when you stumble across a fast-flowing stream. Travelling towards you from the hills, the water sloshes and gurgles, racing past you on its hurried journey to the sea. The monotonous flow of the stream is a soothing escape, an antidote to the fast-paced lives we all lead. The water itself cuts through the land, forming its own path over many years. Observing the body of water voyaging its newfound route, it would be impossible with the naked eye to identify the sum of its parts. Just a mass of substance drifting as one

---

[22] APA. Shilts, R. (2007). And the band played on (20th ed.). St Martin's Press.

homogenous entity, flowing by us as we enjoy the peaceful scene. What we know, from our school science lessons however, is that this is a collective of many individual particles of water. An unimaginable number of H_2O molecules all bumping and colliding together on their merry soiree down to the water table. To put the number of water molecules into context, a standard 500ml bottle of water contains 16.7 septillion H_2O molecules. Yes, '*septillion*' is a thing. It's a thousand raised to the eighth power; or a number with 24 zeros after it.

In the middle of the stream is a raised rock, protruding and sturdy enough to force the water flow to redirect around it. The natural land formation has, unconsciously, found a way to separate the molecules either left or right to then continue their adventure. But wouldn't it be fascinating to learn where all those water molecules had been? Crouching down and scooping a cup of water in your hand, to know if some of the H_2O had circumnavigated the world. Perhaps a few particles had collected on thick waxy leaves in the Amazon rain forest, had spurted out from the blow hole of an Orca in the Atlantic Ocean, once resided deep within a glacier atop a huge mountain in the Himalayas or dramatically plummeted from the Iguazu Falls in South America. In the palm of your hand could be such curious, and well-travelled, water molecules; if only you could separate them out and inspect their credentials in isolation.

That's exactly what they needed for killer blood.

Once a patient received a bone marrow transplant in the 1960s, it was important physicians could monitor the generation of new blood to see if the body was now producing a healthy alternative. Within a few days they would take a sample and try to identify, under the microscope, how many of the blood cells were those of the donor. Was the new bone marrow successfully producing healthy blood and was it doing its job, flowing effectively around the body?

Rather than look at the blood as a collective mass, like the stream, they tried to inspect and sort the individual blood cells under the microscope.

It was a painful process, squinting through the eyepiece for hours at a time, desperate to notice differences and manually separate the blood cells. There must be a better way.

In a cramped and crowded laboratory, in the Department of Genetics of Stanford University, a pair of scientists worked on a solution to the problem. Leonard and Leonore Herzenberg, partners in work and love, were developing a curious new machine that would tag and count all the blood cells much faster and more effectively. Len was getting increasingly frustrated with his deteriorating eyesight and needed a new way to accurately sort and count cells. Leonore, an immunologist from New York, had worked with her husband since they met at Brooklyn College in the early 1950s.

After a time at the Pasteur Institute in Paris, the pair moved to a lab at Stanford University and recognised a need for an automated, high-throughput method to identify individual cells from a population of billions. They created a machine that could count and separate cells in a stream of fluid lit using lasers that revealed fluorescent markers on the cells. Like beekeepers identifying the Queen from the thousands of worker bees using an indicator, but on an altogether vaster scale and at a microscopic level.

What the Herzenberg's had constructed, by 1969, was the fluorescence-activated cell sorter (known as FACS). It had the ability to pick out a single cell in an immense flow of cells; to simultaneously stain, analyse, and then sort those cells based on the markers they were looking for. It provided a method for sorting a mixture of cells into two or more containers, one cell at a time, based upon the specific light scattering and fluorescent characteristics of each cell. As you'd expect when dealing with entities the size of a white blood cell, which is around 20% the width of a human hair[xlvi], the process is somewhat complex[xlvii] but, in short, the invention allowed scientists specialising in immunology to work out the status of the blood cells more efficiently, and in a fraction of the original time, so treatment could begin significantly faster.

This was music to the ears of bone marrow transplantation teams. To be able to quickly mark, sort and analyse the blood cells of a patient could be the difference between life and death; spotting graft failures early and acting, versus missing them leading to disaster.

The FACS invention was one of the greatest advances in clinical and diagnostic immunology and has since been described as the cornerstone of all modern biology. The machines were somewhat expensive but a few leading institutions around the world ordered this first-of-a-kind kit in the 1970s and their scientists started putting them to work. Sometimes the device was used for its intended purpose. Other times it accidentally uncovered what else was really going on.

Serendipitous science

As the symptoms and transmission of the disease became better known, what remained a mystery was how seemingly healthy bodies could succumb. Scientists knew that someone with AIDS had a deficient immune system, disarmed and rendered useless, but what nemesis had done the disarming?

The rise of the new disease (yet to be called AIDS) prompted researchers at the Pasteur Institute in Paris to take a closer look. What if they could jump in before the disease took hold, when patients first experienced symptoms. One such symptom was *lymphadenopathy*, or inflammation of the lymph nodes in the neck. They began searching for answers in the blood, focusing on whether this deadly new disease could be caused by a *retrovirus*.

'Retro', in this context, signifies the virus working backwards; the way the virus propagates its host to thrive. These viruses invade the DNA of a host cell, depositing their own genetics and changing the make-up of the genome. They do this by using an enzyme, known as *reverse transcriptase*, to produce a fake strand of DNA, tricking the original DNA cell into thinking this imitation is, in fact, its own. From then on, the phony genes are recognised as legitimate, accumulating new copies at will.

Dr Francoise Barré-Sinoussi had already been studying retroviruses and leukaemia in mice at the Institute and was familiar with the technique of detecting reverse transcriptase activity. But only one retrovirus was currently known to exist, the human T-lympotropic virus (HTLV), and it could not be that. Taking a lymph node biopsy of a young gay patient with lymphadenopathy, Barré-Sinoussi knew that if she could determine reverse transcriptase activity as present, it would confirm that the cause was a retrovirus.

To investigate Barré-Sinoussi, alongside her colleague Luc Montagnier, used Len and Leonore Herzenberg's fluorescence-activated cell sorting (FACS) machine. It wasn't intended for this use, they'd made it for stem cell procedures, but a bit of shaking, lasering, electrical charges and sorting could identify which blood cells had the hallmarks of a retrovirus. Francoise observed that whatever had infected the patients was actively seeking out and killing the T-cells, or more specifically the CD-4 cells, in the blood stream. They're better known as 'helper cells' because of their crucial role identifying threats and sending signals to other killer cells, like night watchmen, who then attack and destroy. If the CD-4 cells are wiped out there is no one to raise the alarm. By counting the number of CD-4 cells in a 'flow' and determining if this is an expected number or particularly low, it was possible to identify the presence of the adversary in their midst setting about killing them. Finding the retrovirus rampaging and killing immune system cells would allow doctors to determine if a patient would develop AIDS in future.

Barré-Sinoussi identified the culprit; a specific retrovirus, initially called Lymphadenopathy Associated Virus (LAV). They'd used the FACS machine to detect a human immunodeficiency virus that was an unequivocal precursor to AIDS. They'd discovered HIV.

No stone unturned
1974

Pebbles prodded the underside of his feet, cold and wet, as he looked out on the dark and misty seascape. The ocean was black and purple, deep and fearsome, frothing skyward to catch the glint of the moon. Something visible bobbed on the horizon. It moved across, slightly above the vanishing point, back and forth in search of something. Of someone. His legs didn't move; they couldn't. It was a witch. She glided on her broom, dashing the surface, stalking the coast on her hunt. She turned, looking directly at him. He'd been spotted.

Simon woke, sweating. Roger sat beside him, comforting. This dream, the same over and over, was a terror that haunted his nights. There is something we all have in common. Whether a great scientist, athlete, inventor or inspirational world leader. It's something we share with every person that has gone before us. Every person in this book, from famous French double-Nobel Prize winner, Marie Curie, to Dutch textile turned microscope expert, Antoine van Leeuwenhoek, from Canadian Jim Till, the scientist that discovered the stem cell, to mother and accidental campaigner, Liz Bostic.

The universalism of sleep levels us.

During those unconscious hours, when our mind and body recovers and recharges, we are as innocent and vulnerable as a new-born child. Whether snoring, mumbling or silently snoozing, sleep provides a reboot to our immune system. Tissues repair and regrow; the immune response is strengthened and your brain can flush out toxins. Without it, your body remains in stress mode making it easier to get sick.

Liz was vaguely aware of the benefits of sleep. She fixated on creating the optimal environment for Simon; bedtime at 7pm sharp, no sweets or dessert with dinner, the radio and night-light left on to sooth his anxiety. When his night terrors occurred, Roger would dance and play music with Simon to raise a smile, to calm him and encourage happy dreams. Liz had less patience. "Will you just go to sleep" would greet any venture downstairs after dark.

She was less able to control her own sleep pattern. Carrying the guilt of inflicting sickness on her children and balancing the pressures of being an unexpected campaigner in the spotlight she needed help to wind down and dose off. A night cap and sleeping pills. Just enough to weigh heavy on her eyelids, to make her mind fuzzy and calm. It became a habit and it got the job done.

It was during these delirious phases that she weighed up methods of finding a donor. Perhaps a UK tour bus could visit every town and city? What if all NHS staff were compulsorily tested at their job? That could yield a few hundred thousand samples. The fund she'd set up in Andrew's name was raising funds for the Westminster Children's Hospital all the time, bit by bit, to make sure they had the staff and equipment to give kids the best chance of surviving. But she knew there was more they could do. Jack Hobbs explained to Liz, after Simon returned home, "they're dying like flies, it's heart-breaking. It's one thing to watch a child die of an incurable disease, slowly and horribly. Quite another to watch the same thing happening, knowing you have the power to stop it but don't have the means." It all came down to money.

She'd use this pre-sleep time to think what they could have missed. Is there a match out there for everyone? Like a soul mate. For absolutely everyone. If there was – and surely there must be – they simply had to test more people. To find someone to pair with each patient. Record the outcomes in a long-list and see if any match-up with Simon. Like Bingo. For other children, too. Match them off, one by one, until you win a full house.

It was usually at this stage of musing that she drifted off. There was no big picture. The process was a means to an end. Not tonight though. Tonight, she was intent on reading and replying to a handwritten letter she'd received from a woman called Shirley. She was just a year younger than Liz and her son was in a similar position to Simon. Not with the same disease, though. Something instead called Wiskott-Aldrich syndrome, which was incredibly rare apparently. Shirley seemed desperate. She'd already flown her family over from Australia after reading Simon's success story. Quite the risk, Liz thought. But she knew she'd have done the same.

"Just hope and pray and take each day as it comes", Liz advised. "You will be given the strength to carry on. Never give up and never let your mind jump ahead, or else you will start imagining terrible things."

She'd share her ideas of bone marrow bingo with Shirley when they eventually met in-person. Of a list that finds matches for everyone, no matter how rare the blood disease being dealt with. Liz stayed up until 2am writing her response. It's the least she could do to offer some hope.

Shortage of sleep over time led to Liz losing composure. She was short tempered, fits of frantic cleaning would give way to periods of low mood. She began to smoke more. Her fear swelled inside; she'd agitate around Simon, fixating on his every move, his every moment of rest or play. Tolerance of Roger also dwindled. Silent and strong, he may have been battling his own cancer but Liz felt abandoned; fighting demons from all directions, one-handed and unassisted. What Liz didn't know is that Roger felt the same. Did she care if he was there at all?

Simon was a fussy eater. The three-year old would throw unwanted food to the ground if it wasn't to his taste. It tested Liz's patience. Their dog, which wasn't a hygienic choice but due to Liz's love of animals, would gobble whatever it could, sometimes before it reached the ground. The high-level of anxiety that Liz lived with saw her grind through stages of anger, madness and despair with her child.

Simon missed his big brother. He couldn't understand his mother's sadness and sometimes anger. He didn't know how to make his mother happy again. How to make her love him as she had loved Andrew. He felt that he never truly had her attention, even now he was the only child that remained.

Contrastingly, worry for her remaining son was overpowering. Liz developed neurosis for cleanliness and routine and order. For Simon, it was stifling, suffocating, obsessive. It led to limitations in his life. He felt restricted, unable to live like the other children he saw on their walks in the park. He wasn't allowed to play with other children, he couldn't have fun in the mud or adventure on the climbing frame. On a rare occasion he was allowed a playdate with a friend, they bounced on the bed pretending it was a trampoline, seeing which of the pair could reach the highest. Simon fell, smacking his nose against the bedframe and his faulty blood flowed, dyeing the sheets red and prompting hysteria from his mother.

Why was he testing her? She was doing everything in her power to save his life, trying to save even more children's lives, and he still added to her stress. Pat was a local friend and realised Liz was struggling. She was kind and Simon loved spending time with her. She'd sit with him for hours in the kitchen, speaking softly and encouraging him to eat, while Liz took her pills, a Vermouth and slept. Was he riling with intent? He was a central component to what made Liz tick, but he was competing with invisible forces. With Pat he eventually ate. It started with an egg. He was unaware it had been a battle of wills; he was just a fussy eater.

Handing over the baton
1976

"Call me Liz, Shirley. I feel like we know each other well."
Their first meeting, after the numerous letters exchanged, had been friendly and familiar. Shirley found Liz to be a small, intense woman, looking every bit her 28-years, but for whom she had untold respect. It was 1973, sometime in November, and it felt like now was the time to pass on the baton.

Since Simon's transplant in April, Liz's focus had been on recovery and decontamination. Fundraising activity had slowed and, while still running events, the Bostics had achieved their goal. Shirley's quest, however, was only just beginning.

Down to business. The pair discussed the money raised thus far, through the Andrew Bostic Fund, and what they'd been able to spend it on at the Westminster Children's Hospital. So many more transplants, Liz would explain. More technicians employed to tissue type and find matches.

The problem was it needed a heck of a lot more. The bone marrow transplantation department was not completely funded by the NHS, only certain treatments qualified under their remit. Still, despite Simon's world-first transplant, the leading physicians hadn't got the politicians on board. Shirley explained a conversation she'd had with

Jack Hobbs.

"Each transplant', he said, 'costs in the region of £3-4,000. It's expensive, all told. Before a transplant, a child may need blood transfusions of around four-pints per month. These cost £30 per pint so, with that option of spending £1,440 year-on-year, we've shown transplantation can lead to full recovery and no further treatment."

It may have been a little early to predict what longer-term support Simon may need but Hobbs' argument was about false economy. The solution was there but the funding was not.

Doctors called the money they were relying on 'the widow's mite'; smaller than the Government contribution but infinitely more valuable[23]. Liz had worked tirelessly to generate enough money to save her Simon; now it was Shirley's turn.

*

Shirley Nolan was born in Leeds, England, in 1942, and trained as a teacher before emigrating to Darwin, Australia, with her husband James (who she referred to as Ted) in the late 1960s. She was tall, commanding in stature, with a resolute focus of no-nonsense. Typical of the era she let her black, curly hair fall either side of her face, her fringe fell just shy of her eyebrows and when she smiled it was as though you could feel her happiness reach you.

Moving to Adelaide, the couple had their first child in 1971, a little boy called Anthony (pronounced like the 'th' in 'thimble' rather than with a hard 't'?), but it was immediately clear he was not a well little boy. He suffered a catastrophic brain haemorrhage and doctors

---

[23] Reference to the lesson of the widow's mite is presented in Mark 12:41–44, Luke 21:1–4. Someone with comparatively little contributing all they have is more valuable than those with plenty contributing more.

offered little chance of survival. He existed between life and death in hospital and it took his parents eight-months to get him home, by which point he'd been diagnosed with an extremely rare genetic immunodeficiency called Wiskott-Aldrich syndrome.

Named after German paediatrician, Dr Alfred Wiskott, who first identified the disease in 1937, and American paediatrician Dr Robert Anderson Aldrich in 1954, the syndrome is hereditary and mostly impacts male offspring. Similar to CDG, the syndrome that affected the Bostic family, it is a rare inherited X-linked recessive disease, associated with mutations in a gene on the short arm of the X chromosome (Xp11.23), originally termed the Wiskott-Aldrich syndrome protein gene and it is now officially known as WAS (Gene ID: 7454)[xlviii].

Wiskott-Aldrich is a horrific disease, for a number of reasons. Like many blood-related diseases it stops the child's immune system from functioning properly. Not enough operational white cells develop to battle any infection. More than that, though, is the inability of the child's bone marrow to produce platelets; the tiny cell fragments in our blood, shaped just like dinner plates, that form clots to prevent blood escaping outside of our body. This meant the child would be extremely prone to excessive bleeding.

For baby Anthony, the list of symptoms was endless[xlix]. On the outside, his body bruised easily and small spots appeared under the skin's surface, caused by the escape of blood into the tissues from ruptured blood vessels or capillaries. Severe, infected eczema covered his entire body and face, while his eyes swelled and were forced closed with fluid retention[l]. He'd suffer frequent and prolonged nose bleeds, sometimes lasting for hours and needed professional help to stem the flow. Similarly, he'd experience chronic diarrhoea, sometimes for weeks at a time, making him dangerously dehydrated and it was common he would pass blood in his vomit (Hematemesis) or stools (Hematochezia). Most difficult of all for Shirley and James was the knowledge he was always in pain. His external symptoms all considered, what was happening inside his body was arguably far worse.

Lots of internal passageways would swell; his middle ear, airways, sinuses, and large intestine all struggling to function normally under restricted conditions. Not only were there less platelets circulating but fewer red blood cells too. This caused anaemia, meaning oxygen struggled to get around his body and he became fatigued extremely easily. His immune system was dangerously ineffective but he also experienced autoimmunity, meaning the few working immune cells became confused and started attacking his own cells.

Anthony was, in the words of a physician treating him at the time, a "very sick little boy with an incurable disease" and Shirley knew that no child with this diagnosis had lived past three-years. In one unthinkable instance, a doctor told Shirley, "you're wasting your time".

It was the impossible likelihood, and conservative doctors, that made Shirley more determined than ever to prove them wrong.

Reading the news of the young boy, Simon Bostic, in the UK was the glimmer of hope she needed. She immediately called the Westminster Children's Hospital, from her home in Adelaide, and spoke to Jack Hobbs about her son's situation. They'd been led to believe that Shirley's mother was a possible match for Anthony. There was no time to waste. "Professor, Anthony is dying. He's lying in his cot barely breathing. I want to bring him now[24]."

Jack agreed to give it a try. There must be no media around it,

---

[24] Shirley Nolan column, People Magazine

though. The chaos caused in the department by overwhelming public support for Simon had been distracting. What's more, Jack didn't hold out much hope given Anthony's diagnosis. Shirley agreed and booked flights for Anthony and herself to fly to London as soon as possible. He bled the whole way, haemorrhaging and crying for the 36-hour journey to Heathrow where an ambulance picked them up and transferred them directly to the bone marrow transplantation department.

When she stormed through the doors and demanded to sit down with Professor Hobbs and Dr David James, she was physically and emotionally exhausted.

Shirley soon set up camp in a small house in Thanet, a Kent village, just a few hours out of London. It would be their base, their sanctuary, a place for respite in what would become a whirlwind of chaos. They quickly realised that her mother was not a match for Anthony so, with no other family matches, it was back to the drawing board. They would need an unrelated volunteer to come forward. At least now they were in the best place on earth to find a solution.

Treatment yielded slow progress for Anthony. The drugs caused his hair to fall out and his whole body to swell. Like Liz, Shirley felt overwhelmingly helpless so became obsessed with cleanliness, something she *could* control, and days spent at home were saturated with vacuuming and disinfecting. The isolation had an impact on close family ties too. Shirley and her mother's relationship strained, constantly together but never wishing to be apart, they functioned for the greater good. Marital relations suffered worse; Shirley and Ted remained apart, he staying in Adelaide to earn money, but he struggled to accept how much their lives had been turned upside down.

Anthony was admitted to the Westminster Children's Hospital at the end of December 1973. He'd been haemorrhaging relentlessly for days, bleeding from his nose and in his stools, so the professors needed him under observation. Shirley took this opportunity to chat in more detail with Dr David James, the tissue typing guru at the Westminster, whose basement broom cupboard was filling up with blood donations. She couldn't understand why, when all these samples were being received thanks to Liz Bostic's ongoing campaigning, they couldn't find more matches. It was down to funding, he told her. They could tissue type up to 50 samples every day with two technicians, he explained, but funding had been withdrawn. They needed £3,000.

Shirley instantly sprang into action. Against their advice she broke the agreed media ban and took to the streets. She'd talk to anyone that listened; she promoted her campaign outside school gates, at churches, at people's homes. Often found holding vigil outside the Palace of Westminster, Shirley and friends would wave placards and attempt to commandeer politicians to help them understand her plight. On one occasion she protested a little too passionately, being detained by the police for disturbing the peace. In typical Shirley fashion, the incident resulted in numerous Metropolitan Police officers signing up to donate their bone marrow.

Unlike Liz, who had stumbled into campaigning, Shirley was acute in her objectives. She'd raise money for a technician, explaining that her boy's life was at stake. More than that, she would amalgamate all this DNA data, establishing a clear, searchable registry of donor tissue type data to make more unrelated matches possible. To find that needle in a haystack for Anthony, and others like him. Liz Bostic had vocalised the need to explore this further, Shirley was really the first person in the world to plan a structured organisation to collect data, made available for people suffering from leukaemia and other killer blood diseases on a voluntary basis[li].

Within a few months, four technicians crammed into that tiny basement broom cupboard. Shirley's campaigning had hit home and public money was coming in. Around the same time, in 1974, the Anthony Nolan appeal for donors was officially founded. Behind the scenes and always supportive, Liz watched as Shirley took the concept of unrelated bone marrow transplants to a new level. Writing human interest features in women's magazines was Liz's way of raising awareness now, telling her family's story, but also encouraging Shirley's tireless frontline campaigning. "She was my greatest ally", Shirley would go on to say.

Progress was painfully slow for Anthony himself. No matched donor was found and his health fluctuated over the coming years. He'd spend long periods in hospital, at times just hours away from death, yet would rally to return home with his mother to the clean, countryside air of rural Kent. It was a tough routine, often beginning at 4am. If he was haemorrhaging, something that was a weekly occurrence, it could last for seven-hours. It took all Shirley and her mother's energy to calm Anthony, cold-compresses on his head, singing to relax him, keeping him warm. They lived in absolute isolation. The three of them, cut off from the viruses and unknowns of the outside world, setting out on this lonely, daily challenge. It was something Liz had warned Shirley about. The feeling of remoteness, unable to connect with other around who want to give support.

In 1976, the bone marrow donor registry officially became a charity; The Anthony Nolan Bone Marrow Appeal. It was the first stem cell register in the world.

Never before had genetics been stored on a register in the hope of matching with a stranger. Shirley designed the logo, making sure it included an eight-petalled daisy, signifying that we all consist of lots of parts and, even if one is removed, we fundamentally remain who we are. Up to 100 tests were taking place every week meaning that at any time, literally any day, a donor might be found for Anthony.

They came excruciatingly close. On a chance trip to New Zealand, Dr James discovered that the blood of a trainee medical technician was the same tissue type as Anthony. Samoan, Malo Ioane, could be that unrelated match and, within three-days, he was sitting in the Westminster Hospital donating his stem cells. He'd never travelled before but had been motivated to cross the world to try and save an unknown baby's life.

It was almost unbelievable for Shirley. Years of raising awareness, cajoling doctors and caring for her child could soon be over. Since she began, five children had received transplants thanks to the register. She hoped Anthony's could be the sixth.

Six days they had to wait. Testing took place in culture, introducing Malo's stem cells to Anthony's in a dish, to see how compatible they were. "We're very, very sorry but it's no good', Dr James explained gently, in his soft Welsh accent, 'Anthony's cells have rejected those of Mr Ioane." It was devastating news. Shirley didn't crumble into a heap of tears but retained her public face, thanking the doctors. Secretly she was overwhelmed by numbness. Her weariness and unknown future for Anthony left her utterly depressed. There was no end to it. But she felt responsible, not only for Anthony's life but also for the lives of hundreds of other children all over the world because the register was now open to other countries. She had to find the will to carry on.

One afternoon when the pair met for tea, Shirley told Liz she couldn't take any more bad news. She wanted to end it all; false hope had become her only diet, she simply didn't know how she could accept more setbacks and continue fighting to keep Anthony alive. "I don't know how you keep going', Liz told her, 'but don't stop."

Big data to solve a big problem
1980s

The social worker sat balanced on the edge of the hospital bed, twisting to face Laura whose hand she securely cradled within her own. A silent moment between the pair. A sustained look as Laura processed the news. The conversation, delicate as it had been, referred to her own mortality. That now, despite it all, it was probable she would die.

After a few seconds, and without diverting her gaze, Laura responded: "just don't tell my mommy."

Two years later, lying in her parents' king-size bed at their home in northern Colorado, Laura continued to explain that her daddy would figure something out. Her hero had already achieved so much and she knew he would stop at nothing. His ear was fixed to the phone, his face forever frowning, it seemed like he didn't sleep.

Laura's blood disease had led scientists to search far and wide for a bone marrow match. With local options exhausted, physicians and researchers knew a solution would have to be found further afield. They needed to collaborate with other institutions across the United States, ask them to share all their transplant outcomes data, both good and bad. An idea easier said than done.

The morphine machine rattled next to her pillow while oxygen pumped into the mask fixed over her nose and mouth. But her body had reached the intersection. And Laura knew it. As the afternoon sun snook through the window blinds, her parents either side and reading a story, 12-year-old Laura proposed her last idea: "nothing is working, mom. Let's try some chicken soup."

Sea dogs teaching us new tricks

Gawping out of a grocery store window in the small Yorkshire fishing village of Staithes, a teenage apprentice called James Cook daydreamed of adventurous exploration. Each day he'd keenly observe the ebb and flow, ripple and crash of the ocean before him and, as months slowly passed in his first ever job, his mind wandered to possibilities of what existed beyond the mystical line where the waves met the sky. Imagination captured by the majesty of the sea, stirred by colourful folklore of local fishermen he'd meet, he won an apprenticeship with a merchant sailing company and set out boldly to find his way on the water, intent on discovery.

He was 26 when he finally joined the Royal Navy, quickly rising through the ranks and 'Lieutenant' Cook was soon commissioned to lead an expedition of important scientific discovery to the Pacific Ocean. It was 1769 and his maiden voyage in command. While science was part of the remit, namely observing the Transit of Venus across the surface of the Sun in the ongoing quest to solve the Longitude problem, the primary objective (only revealed to him in full while already at sea) was to search for a hypothetical continent believed to be somewhere in the South Hemisphere. That of 'Terra Australis'. Navigating past what is now New Zealand, Cook's ship, the HMS Endeavour, reached the east coast of Australia in April 1770, becoming the first Europeans to dock on the land. The following months led to exciting explorations of the eastern coast, sailing north from their initial landing in 'Stingray Bay', which he later renamed Botany Bay, the crew documented everything from botanical discoveries to tentative (read: 'hostile') encounters with aboriginal natives.

It was 10th June 1770 when the Endeavour encountered a serious problem. At 11pm, around one hour after passing Pickersgill Reef, they "struck on a reef of coral" and ran aground; a razor-sharp stretch of rocks that will later be known as the Great Barrier Reef. Cook and his crew had woefully misjudged the tide. On this occasion there was no loss of life; it was more embarrassing than anything else with the hull severely damaged. The local Guugu Yimithirr tribe watched as the ship limped to shore, docking at the mouth of the river, known locally as Wahalumbaal. Travels were put on hold for around seven weeks while extensive repairs were carried out.

Cook was, however, perplexed. How had his tidal calculations gone so amiss. Determined to show his superiors that this wasn't simply inexperience, he focused his gaze this time from the window of his private quarters onboard. With the cackling of pebbles his soundtrack, shuffling and resettling with the waves, Cook set about meticulously documenting the tidal water marks in the bay; like a parent scoring pencil lines on the kitchen wall to denote height changes of a child. Cook observed that the neap tides (when tide is at its minimum) were significantly lower than the spring tide (when tide is at its maximum; 'spring' meaning leap or jump, rather than the season). His notes show that the 'spring tides rose by nine feet perpendicularly in the evening, and scarcely seven [feet] in the morning'. During weeks of observation from his stricken vessel he noted that the difference was uniformly the same over the series of spring tides.

He was confused but, in his writings, entitled 'On the Tides of the

South Seas', Cook said "he leaves it for others to supply the explanation".

Getting caught out by the tide was an occupational hazard for seafarers. Even the most skilled and experienced sea dogs, as in the case of the now heralded explorer Captain James Cook, were sometimes caught off-guard by the tide.

So, what changed – and what has this adventurous tale got to do with blood disease? It's all to do with learning from observation and sharing data.

We didn't always know about the behaviour of the ocean.

Theories about tides and their relationship with the moon date back over 2,000 years. Ancient fishermen and mariners developed simple prediction methods based on the observed time interval between the moon's highest ascent above the horizon and the next high water. They also knew that the tidal range varied throughout the month, increasing as one approached full or new moon. For the most part, however, it was pretty much guess work.

The first physical oceanographic data series was probably the tabulation of the times and heights of high and low waters at the northern end of the Persian Gulf, compiled around 150 BC by the Hellenistic mathematician Seleucus of Babylon. Seleucus recognized that the two high tides on any given day could be quite different in height and that the difference varied throughout the month, being greatest when the moon is farthest north or south of the equator[25].

Other notable theorists came much later, including Persian Muslim astrologer Abu Ma'shar in 886 and German astrologer Johannes Kepler in the earlier 1600s. Yet it wasn't until an apple fell from a

---

[25] Tide Predictions for D-Day, Bruce Parker: Physics Today 64, 9, 35 (2011); doi: 10.1063/PT.3.1257

tree and collided with the head of English mathematician Isaac Newton, and he published his equilibrium theory in *Principia* in 1687, that someone explained tides as the product of the gravitational attraction of astronomical masses.

Misjudging the tide often proved a costly business so great efforts and investments were made to better predict timings. Arguably the most important of these was by William Thompson in the 1860s. Further developing the theories of Newton, Belfast-born Thompson introduced the harmonic analysis for tidal observations, building a super-computer (of sorts) which could predict the tides on any given day using an arithmetic formula based on energy and trigonometry. The mathematical physicist's ingenious machine, complete with greasy pullies, clunky gears and moveable brass shafts, was connected to a pen which scribbled on paper to record the frequency. Those energies vary from place to place because of the way oceans, bays, and other waterways affect the tide. But the brilliance of the harmonic method was that it required no expert understanding of hydrodynamics. One simply needed to record and analyse a long-enough data set at each location to create fairly accurate predictions.

Using this genius machine, tide predictions were made for an entire year for all major ports and harbours around the world for which figures had been taken (usually requiring around one-years' worth of 'big' data). As the years passed the basic harmonic method changed relatively little with the transition to digital computers; numerical equations and high-tech kit just replaced the pulleys and gears.

Thompson later became Lord Kelvin and we still measure absolute temperatures in units of 'kelvin' in his honour. His machines stood the test of time, even having a significant impact on the outcome of

World War II.[26]

If you go to your nearest coast today, you'll find high tide time predictions to the nearest minute, sometimes nonchalantly scratched onto a chalk board. That accuracy is not finger-in-the-air guesswork, as we have seen, but advancements on our ability to predict 'ebb and flow' starting 2,000 years ago by observing the moon through to mathematical formulas in the last 350 years. These are then published and widely shared to make sure others do not fall foul of changing tides, like Captain Cook.

Since this time, large data sets have been used and shared by sailors for hundreds of years. By contrast, the medical world was a long way behind, yet to find a way of collecting best-practice. This was about to change.

Sharing data in medicine

When Laura Graves died it was exactly five-years to the day after her first treatment for leukaemia. Another child gone; another family left utterly bereft.

The news of Laura's death delivered a seismic blow to the team at the Fred Hutchinson Cancer Research Center in Seattle. She was the first leukaemia patient in the U.S. to receive a bone marrow transplant from a non-related donor, six-years after Simon Bostic in London, a momentous procedure of such promise as her recovery

---

[26] In 1944, Prime Minister, Winston Churchill asked the Admiralty for "a chart of the tides and moons to cover the next six weeks" to determine "on which days conditions will be most favourable for a seaborne landing". Using Kelvin's machine, the British opted for an audacious low-tide attack and calculated that Normandy was the ideal spot along the coast. The accuracy of tidal predictions, based on the collection of big data, enabled the D-Day landings, possibly one of the pivotal moments in the Allied advance against Nazi occupied France.

had led her back into school and to a 'normal' way of life. But more than that the team had become deeply invested in Laura as a person. None more so than young immunologist, John Hansen.

Minnesotan Dr Hansen joined The Hutch in 1977, not long after it had opened its doors, at a time when bone marrow transplantation was experimental, last-ditch and, predominantly, not working. Light-brown hair combed in a side parting, large glasses covering half his face, 34-year-old John Hansen was excitable about an area of medicine on the cusp of great things. He'd previously fancied a career focused on heart transplantation but, by chance, ended up working at the University of Minnesota with Dr Robert Good: the specialist responsible for the first successful bone marrow transplant between siblings in 1968. Learning from such an esteemed colleague, who's excitement was contagious, and Dr Hansen completely switched paths, ending up in Seattle.

In his new role he focused primarily on finding suitable bone marrow matches for patients; comparing the tissue type (HLA) to that of potential donors knowing that the closer they matched the more likely the success rate. He meticulously gathered his data, logging it all on coloured prompt cards, filing in a binder and storing in a locked lab cabinet. When his colleague, lab technician Frances Otto-Depner, appeared as a near perfect match for Laura Graves, he immediately knew this was the best chance they'd ever seen to try their experimental, and risky, first unrelated transplantation.

For the gamble to pay off, Hansen needed to meticulously study big data sets. In this instance, the bigger the better, so he'd built close ties with the newly formed *Center for International Blood and Marrow Transplant Research (CIBMTR)* in the neighbouring state of Wisconsin, led by Dr Mortimer (Mort) Bortin. Officially set up in 1972, but collecting outcomes of transplants since 1970, this new unit was possibly the first-time big data was seen as a tool to improve medical treatment. The programme intended to collect and analyse outcomes of transplants from across the U.S. all in one place, from all 12 transplant centres, but it was a bold ambition. People don't naturally like to share details of failure and, at this time, outcomes were predominantly failures. The CIBMTR managed to encourage open and transparent data sharing unheard of in medical circles to that point. Dr Mort Bortin, the mastermind, knew that there was no substitute for observation. Only by seeing all possible outcomes from transplants across the country could they grasp trends that would improve treatment. It was a treasure trove of learning to immunologists and, as the years progressed, this insight outcome data set simply grew exponentially.

Laura's legacy

For John Hansen, an impromptu meeting in a hospital hallway got the ball rolling. Laura's father, Bob, walked to grab a coffee at the machine when Dr Hansen intercepted him. He wanted to discuss the option of the transplant.

The previous two gruelling years of chemotherapy, which she started at the age of 10, had been tough: radiation sickness, painful side effects of drugs included a swollen face and hands, and the loss of her hair made her return to school, and the lack of understanding from her classmates, particularly hard.

But while Laura was believed to be in 'remission', a temporary abeyance of the symptoms, tests revealed that the leukaemia cells had come back; she had relapsed. This form of treatment wasn't working, Hansen explained to Bob, and no patient had ever recovered once the leukaemia returned. The only remaining treatment option was a bone marrow transplant: to replace Laura's ineffective immune system with a new one to fight off the disease.

Hansen explained that behind-the-scenes for the last seven years, he and Don Thomas had been considering the option of matching with a non-relative donor. They'd never done it before, and it posed an obvious risk, but if all three of Laura's siblings returned dissimilar tissue types, he asked if the family would consider receiving the bone marrow of a stranger?

The question was hypothetical. Hansen knew the siblings were not matched but that an almost identical match had *already* been found. He'd give the family time to think it over, but this first-of-a-kind experiment in the United States may be Laura's only chance.

Bob's response in the hallway was swift, "Yes, please look into that option, but don't tell my wife". It seems father and daughter shared a common goal to protect Sherry.

Laura's transplant, on 4th September 1979, was deemed a success. The engraftment had 'taken', which meant the donated cells (the graft) took root in the bone marrow and began to make healthy new red blood cells, white blood cells and platelets. The transfusion had taken place intravenously, through the department's pioneering 'Hickman Line' catheter, and she spent the next 90-days recovering in the germ-free laminar air flow room – otherwise known as 'the bubble' – to allow her new immune system to form. News spread of the ground-breaking transplant and, as she 'celebrated' her 11th birthday inside the bubble, Laura received messages, cards and toys from family and friends back in Colorado plus a few from celebrities too, John Travolta, Burt Reynolds and Sally Field among those that sent 'get well' messages.

She hated that bubble. Nothing could get inside unless it had been radiated first to ensure no germs crossed the boundary. Laura's schoolteacher didn't miss a beat, getting some textbooks blasted and into her hands.

It all paid off and that Christmas Laura was back home in Fort

Collins. Everyone took care to wear masks and clean surfaces but, when January came around, it was time for a well-deserved family trip to Disneyland.

Laura's dad, Bob Graves, was a farmer, the fourth generation of a dairy and ranching family in northern Colorado. His wife Sherry fondly called him the last frontier man of the Old West: rugged, stubborn, blunt, with a driven work ethic. He ran the family's farm and the dairy store they owned in Bellevue, just outside of Fort Collins. He didn't, he'd openly admit, know much about immunology, haematology or transplantation. But that wasn't going to stop him dedicating the rest of his life to a new venture in partnership with the world's leading scientists in those specialisms.

After Laura's bone marrow transplant, Bob received calls and messages from parents across the United States desperate to learn how they could find a donor. Their child, like Laura those months ago, was seemingly helpless as death flagrantly edged closer each day and, hearing of this first-of-a-kind experimental transplant, gave them fresh hope. So, Bob set up a makeshift office in his basement and, after a day of farming, he'd retreat down in an evening to help other families find a match. At the time, around 60% of all patients needing a life-saving transplant did not have a family member match and Bob, pragmatic as ever, started calling all the blood banks across the country to learn if they were capturing the HLA type of their donors. The answer was predominantly 'no' and, when he'd occasionally find a match for a child against the odds, he'd call the family only to be told that the patient was already dead. It needed to be centralised. To be fast and reactive. The answer would involve creating an open network that could identify potential matches instantly. Some sort of accessible registry, within which each entry could potentially save a life.

While plans started to take shape, Laura's health again spiralled towards the end of 1980 and, a year after transplantation, the leukaemia had returned. Always a man of action, Bob convened a meeting of leading scientists, doctors, blood bank staff, patients and donors for a meeting to discuss the need for a donor registry in Denver in March 1981. Laura attended, as did Dr Hansen who flew over from Seattle. Hansen understood the potential of a network approach to the tissue typing. To collect the sample, to share the data, and incrementally perfect the degree of accuracy would improve the survival chances of bone marrow transplantation patients everywhere. It could even save lives around the world. But this would take huge investment and, with little evidence this method was working, none was forthcoming. Even though the engraftment had proved that an unrelated donor could be used, Laura's health was in devastating decline. Despite no funding, researchers at CIMBTR continued to inspect outcomes data from transplant centres, and *The Laura Graves National Bone Marrow Transplant Foundation* was born.

In a final throw of the dice in July 1981, Bob, Sherry and Laura all boarded a plane to London.

Bob made it his job to read anything and everything about bone marrow transplantation and the pioneering work of the Westminster Children's Hospital came up time and again. Specifically, Bob had made a plan to speak with Dr David James and Professor Jack Hobbs, the architects, as far as he could gather, of the programme in London. There must be one last chance for Laura, he thought, and this team had created the first ever registry of donors in the world a few years before[27]. Could there be a *new* match for Laura? The news wasn't what they'd hoped for. A second dose of full body

---

[27] The Anthony Nolan Bone Marrow Registry, in 1974

irradiation for Laura was deemed too risky. As they left Dr James' new laboratory at St Mary Abbots Hospital in London, they knew that a second transplant was off the table. She just wouldn't survive the ordeal.

Less than a month later, when Sherry returned to the king-sized bed with the bowl of steaming chicken soup, Laura had died.

The omnipresence of mortality had stalked the Graves' for many years, each day they felt consumed by purposeful evasion. It required a concerted effort to inject hope, banishing the lurking darkness from the front of the mind. Yet Laura's death turned that darkness into a black hole which threatened to drag in those left behind unless they filled it quickly. Sherry transferred her attention to her other three children, aware that uneven attentiveness needed balancing. Bob doubled his energies toward Laura's legacy by refocusing on the idea of a registry. Perhaps encouraged by what he'd seen in London at the Anthony Nolan Bone Marrow Registry, he dedicated himself night and day to advocating for investment in this life-saving network.

Bob stayed in close contact with Don Thomas and John Hansen at The Hutch but his hopes of a national bone marrow registry kept hitting snags. The primary snag being that no one was interested.

As he bullishly continued his personal pursuit in the coming years from the basement of his home, the politicians and lawmakers simply refused to invest in a treatment that was yet to yield sufficient unequivocal merit. There was no political will and, therefore, no funding.

The team at The Hutch left him to it, full of praise for his typical resilient rancher approach but unable to afford him too much of their time. That was until a letter from the American Red Cross arrived in the mailbox on his lawn inviting him to a joint meeting at the University of Minnesota, in Minneapolis. The message that asked Bob to attend, alongside Thomas and Hansen, had been a little cryptic. Why, suddenly, were people interested? Had his uncompromising campaigning finally been heard?

As the meeting date approached, Bob and Sherry watched a report on the ABC World News Tonight about the unusually high numbers of U.S. military, returned from active service ten-years prior, that were now being diagnosed with, and dying from, cancer.

Unbeknownst to Bob, still a humble farmer in rural Colorado, this military predicament would soon enter his reality and see him join forces with someone who was every bit as uncompromising as himself.

Another life over too soon
1978

Standing over the lifeless body of her child she felt a gut-twisting clench, and she wept. Reaching down she lifted a pale hand into her own, cocooning it, cold and unresponsive, but still the hand of her child. No parent should outlive their children. Your baby is dead, a verdict worse than your own death. After years of torment, so much endured, everything achieved. It was a cruel jest.

The hospital called as soon as they had realised. A moment of silence through the receiver before the whimpers could be heard. To have died alone, without comfort or solace, is something a parent that brought a human into the world cannot simply come to terms with. She thought back to childhood, cradling her new-born against her bosom, those first tentative steps, the first garbled words.

Resting the hand gently back in place on the bed, delicately stroking hair away from the eyes, Mollie felt her tears cascade, falling from her cheeks onto her daughter below.

Liz didn't deserve this, her mother Mollie thought. After years of campaigning, the terror of losing a child and the struggle to save another. Perhaps the spectre haunting her never left. Maybe it was only ever a matter of time before she reunited with her Andrew. Or what if it was simply a mistake, a fit of fury, an error of judgement? She'd known the risk. To dangle with intent so close to the edge, to allow yourself to peer over the void yet expect to escape the drop. Liz just needed to take a break from it all; to flee, even if only for a little while. As Simon, now seven-years-old, recovered nearby in the Westminster Children's Hospital from worrying new symptoms, he would soon discover that his mother had died.

He would never see her again.

*

And so, to the denouement of this tortuous piece.

Almost 80-years prior, Edith Mond had found the trials of caring for dying children a worry too heavy to bear. She'd dedicated her life to building a place of safety, comfort and love so that infants, and their families, could live out their final moments privately and in peace. All those years ago she'd also longed for momentary release, from the suffering, the hospital wards, the noise of distressed infants and the constant reality of mortality around each corner. The tablets she'd taken were to escape the trial; assumed responsibility for the children dying that she, and Dr Vincent, were unable to save.

The hospital built in her honour was now the scene of a new tragedy. A similar momentary lapse, perhaps. A strangely similar coincidence, for sure. After 10-years of torturous dread, and just a year older than Edith had been, it was all over for Liz.

There's solemn little else to add, really. A mother of two young boys battled to save them from an internal demon and almost certain death. She succeeded with one of them. That, itself, was incredible. She was the first parent in history, given this prognosis, to ever achieve a successful outcome for their child.

The order of events is a luckless affair. Simon had ominously been admitted back into hospital suffering with high fevers, night sweats and a suspicious pain in his shoulder when inhaling. After these glorious infection-free years of reprieve, Liz knew it was starting all over again. Simon saw her noticeably agitated and scared. It must have all come flooding back; the pressures, the press, the relentless probing, puncturing and probabilities. With Simon settled in the familiar cold and sterile cubicle, Liz asked a matron for the key to the Mother's Unit; she longed for a lie-down and a cigarette.

"There are no rooms available for you to use at the moment. I can quickly set up a Z-bed for you in Simon's cubicle otherwise you'll have to just leave him here with us." The matron's words ignited a blaze of claustrophobic fear and venomous fury. The prospect of the grey metallic bedframe, sickly plastic mattress and hostile cubicle walls left her feeling trapped, like a caged animal. But she'd not leave her baby here alone. He needed her. On this sweaty and stifling July day she longed for the calming green room, the private escape to call her friend and to chat and offload and smoke. She was willing to fight for it, for her safe space; her toil had earned it. Roger did not understand. She was overreacting, he'd say. They must remain calm, he'd insist.

Simon's legs dangled from the bed as his parents engaged in word-warfare before him, a scene from battle as the insults flung back and forth like gunfire until the heat, pressure and decibel levels in the room seemed like they could shatter windows. Everyone on the ward saw it, those that didn't certainly heard it. Then no more words. Simon fixated on the rhythmic swish of his mother's skirt as she flung open the door and charged away down the deserted corridor. Her flame red hair spewed like lava, the melodic clunk of her heels a haunting soundtrack to her exit from Simon's life.

What happened next was not entirely unprecedented for Liz. At these increasingly frequent moments of overwhelming stress, she find solace with a dose of prescribed tranquilisers and anti-depressants. Momentary release from the pressures. It had almost come to this before, of course. Liz had once taken too many tranquilisers and needed to have her stomach pumped. She'd explained to a furious Mollie, "I wasn't thinking – I just needed to get away from it all for a while." This occasion was different. As her friend heard Liz's voice trail away on the other end of the receiver, Roger walked into the room and saw Liz's faded frame, semi-conscious, collapsed on the green carpet. "It's alright Rodge, I've taken more of the other ones this time". Instead of taking a few extra tranquilizers to help her calm down, she'd taken more anti-depressants, lethal at high doses.

Liz had wanted a moment of rest, to ease the tension, but surely never intentionally abandoned Simon. It was probably unintentional but it was her own mistake.

Liz was kept alive in a coma for a little over two-weeks. She existed without existing.

One day, Roger walked Simon across Vincent Square for some fresh air. They walked from the Children's Hospital to a little park outside the adult unit where, five-floors up in the ICU, Liz was being kept alive. Simon craned his neck skyward, squinting at the gloomy-looking building. Roger explained that mummy was sleeping and nurses were looking after her. He avoided answering Simon's question, "will she wake up, daddy?".

Simon was never allowed to visit her properly. He didn't understand. Deep down he had a feeling he'd never see her again. He wasn't allowed to say goodbye. As his own health quickly improved, with pleurisy the eventual diagnosis, he craved the touch of his mother's hand one last time.

It wasn't to be. His mum was gone. Losing a parent, no matter at what age, digs deep at the core of a person. For a boy of just seven, who's life had been filled with pain, grief and anxiety, the rug was completely pulled from under him. His world emptied.

Simon's final mental image was painful; Liz fighting with Roger, storming away down the hospital corridor and the silent, swinging door closing shut behind her. A painful imprint that remains forever. What if a bed had been available? What if he hadn't become sick? He felt entirely responsible.

The next morning the Daily Express frontpage read, "Tragedy of a loving mother" with a photo of Liz, Roger and Simon. Two weeks after her death, the money she had been raising to support treatment at the Westminster Children's Hospital sprang into life. The machine her funding paid for – which cost £250 each day to run – was keeping a four-year old girl alive after her recent bone marrow transplant. Dr David James was quoted in the newspaper as saying they could be doing these life-saving operations twice-monthly if they had the funds but, instead, they could only afford to do one. Without a transplant, as Simon had had five-years before, the children would almost certainly die. Without the newly renamed Andrew and Elisabeth Bostic Fund, transplants would become a thing of the past at the hospital.

The coroner recorded, "this is not the usual calm and settled intent of suicide". No one believed she did it on purpose. The papers claimed she died of a love that could take no more[lii].

Not only did she transform it in life but her death had another immediate impact in the world of transplantation. Her liver and kidneys were used within a week to give hope to patients in Liverpool and London, but the register she began – almost without realising it – would have global impact beyond what even she could have envisaged.

Liz's death sparked a new wave of press attention. The Daily

Express newspaper continued their support, setting up a trust fund for Simon to their readers with the headline, "No, Simon will not walk alone", and money came flooding in from across the country. They wanted to give this young boy the best chance in life. Tabloid headlines exclaimed that his mother died through a drug overdose and feared he could be orphaned – Roger was still being treated for lung cancer. Readers were encouraged to help this 'impish little miracle' to have a shot at life.

Shirley Nolan recalled her recent catch-up with Liz. "I don't know how you keep going', Liz told her, 'but don't stop."

Those were the last words Liz ever said to Shirley.

On hearing the news of her premature death, during a brief family break back in Australia, Shirley sent flowers to the hospital: "To Liz, With love from Anthony and Shirley, half the world away. Our prayers are with you." In a letter to Mollie, a few months later, she explained, "Liz did not die in vain and will forever be alive in my heart."

Liz's death initiated a flurry of financial donations. Landing back in the UK, it was full steam ahead for Shirley and the hospital professors. In September 1978, just two months later, the Anthony Nolan laboratories opened at St Mary's Abbot Hospital. No more cramped working in a basement broom cupboard. These were specifically designed labs for tissue type testing and indexing of volunteer donors. In 1978, at the time of Liz's death, over 17,000 people had signed up to the registry.

The beginning of Elisabeth Bostic's legacy.

Scientists worked diligently but never found a match for Anthony. Just over a year later, on 21st October 1979, his short and difficult life was over. Aged just seven years old, much older than his prognosis but far too young all the same, Shirley said a painful goodbye to Anthony, her only child.

"I cannot realise as yet Anthony's death", she explained to Liz's mother, Mollie, in a private letter just one-month later. "He had such a vital personality that I can still feel him all around me. I do know that I must continue to try to help others (as your dear Elisabeth did) so that Anthony's short life will not have been meaningless."

That spirit, to continue relentlessly through grief, is a trait both Shirley and Liz possessed. Their moment in time, and pursuit of progress, laid foundations for life-saving treatment across the world. Those suffering fatal blood disease would look to the work and attitude of these women for rescue, wherever they may live and whatever may have caused their circumstance.

Life changed dramatically for Simon after his mother's death[28].

He was seven and felt the loss heavily. He felt the grief surrounding him. He wasn't allowed to attend his mother's funeral or memorial service and couldn't understand why. It was his fault she had died, he decided. If he hadn't been admitted to hospital his mother would still be here. He blamed himself.[29]

"Dear friends, thank you very much for my presents. Love Simon Bostic".

The photographer captured Simon in deep concentration, hunched up on a wooden park bench writing a letter to the readers of the Daily Express as he left hospital just weeks after Liz's death. He was being discharged, heading home for the first time, and it was an opportunity to express the family's gratitude for such public

---

[28] Bostic, Simon: The Marrow of Life (blog), http://www.themarrowoflife.com/2019/08/that-day-in-july/comment-page-1/#comment-39

[29] Simon's blamed himself, just as Liz had blamed her genetics for passing on the defect and Mollie felt she must have been responsible for Liz being a carrier of CGD.

affection and support. Over $50,000 had been donated to the Andrew and Elisabeth Bostic Fund, sufficient to supply the Westminster Children's Hospital with staff and equipment to support many more children in similar situations to Simon.

Two-weeks later, Roger and Simon flew to Malta. An anonymous donor paid for the trip to allow the family to recover; to bring stability at the end of the rocky road. They spent time by the swimming pool, his father chatted with other adults as Simon played in the water. An unlooked for consequence of this holiday was Roger meeting a young women whom he came to hope would help him raise his motherless boy. It was so soon.

Exactly one-year after Liz's death and the Westminster Children's Hospital, that saved Simon's life, was also on the brink of collapse.

The Government had told them, and all hospitals, to tighten their belts meaning one of the wards would be forced to close. Jack Hobbs didn't waste a minute. He was determined that his department wouldn't get the chop. He went against all guidance and invited a journalist to visit the ward, meet the children and families, and publish a story about the bone marrow transplantation work being the most important in the building. It didn't go down well inside Udall Street, but Jack didn't much care. His priority was always bone marrow transplants; his colleagues should have been as single-minded as him, he'd say. An appeal to Daily Express readers to save more children, like Simon, ensuring Government ministers couldn't ignore him.

He also asked the Bostic's to return the publicity favour, this time talking to the media to save his department. Simon and Roger chatted to reporters with notepads and video cameras, their faces and words appearing on televisions and newsstands across the country. Around the same time, Simon, now aged eight, stood above the train tracks near his home. It was becoming too much. Survivor guilt never left him when he remembered his brother, Andrew. More so when he remembered his mum. If only he'd been able to stay healthy, or at least keep pretending. He'd lost half of the people he loved and felt alienated from his replacement family. He needed to escape. Despite his young age, he meant it. Looking down from the bridge at the train tracks he thought of his Nanny and decided to go home. He told no one.

Sometime later, Mollie took Simon in and he went to secondary school as a boarder, thanks to the Daily Express fund. There he met new friends, found new opportunities and enjoyed a stable and caring environment. It provided the space for recovery he so desperately needed to transition to adulthood.

Attempts to right so many wrongs
mid-1980s

A deep thudding chuff-chuff surfed the Delta as harmonised propellers soundtracked the majestic formation sweeping the horizon. Trailing a delicate mist, like a laced flowing bridal train, the triad of helicopters moved as one; theatrical players in a split-screen scene of green and blue. Colourless vapour glided from extended arms, silently graceful in descent through the early morning sky. Like a tide crashing at shore, a sprawling wall of liquid plunged to an almighty crescendo, pummelling thick waxy leaves in a synchronised smack.

On a day bright, harsh with sun, any woodland or forest offers a cooling oasis of respite. Fallen branches crack underfoot, rich smells seep and birds sing. A canopy of plants and leaves shield a darkened underworld of ecological mysteries; the perfect setting for an expansive contest of hide and seek.

The U.S. President, John F. Kennedy, however, wasn't in a position to entertain the long game.

His political advisors compared the situation to his wasted hours as an amateur golfer searching aimlessly for stray balls hidden among the thick, uncut grass lining the fairway. Imagine, they explained, you could miraculously disappear all that wretched greenery of overgrown rough. In one stroke vanish the source of concealment, to reveal only your glistening ball, invitingly positioned on a perfect lie, primed and unhindered to resume your progress to the hole. It was an analogy Kennedy enthusiastically understood. The *real* game was the Vietnam War. The hidden golf ball the Việt Cộng; a guerrilla movement supporting North Vietnam interests. And the wondrous tool for removing the overgrown bush, Agent Orange.

A little background, first. A few years beforehand in the Malaya conflict of the 1950s, British armed forces tactically deployed a chemical herbicide to destroy enemy food crops grown in inaccessible parts of the jungle. A new way to hit them where it hurts. Widespread concerns that this was 'chemical warfare' were dismissed as the British stated these herbicides were "harmless to human and animal life". Despite this convenient assertion, this use of herbicides breached the Geneva Convention and international law. There were, however, no international repercussions - they got away with it - and a precedent was set.

Following the Brits lead, *Operation Ranch Hand* commenced in early 1962. This was the large-scale destruction of bushes, crops and trees of the various Deltas in Vietnam to expose and thwart the Việt Cộng tactics of using the dense foliage as cover when ambushing nearby U.S. military. Spraying a range of chemical agents named, 'Rainbow Herbicides', the plan was to severely reduce capacity for rural land dwellers to produce their own food, including Việt Cộng fighters, which would force them to migrate out of the jungle. The chief weed killer of the bunch was Agent Orange.

Before all this, the U.S. had opted to support former colonisers France in the South when Vietnam split, in July 1954, mainly as leader Hồ Chí Minh and the Communist North were believed to be financially backed by the Soviet Union and the People's Republic of China. Threatened by the West's perceived expansion of Communism, known as The Red Scare, stability in Vietnam took on greater global significance to the President.

For most of 1962, the first year of the Ranch Hand operation, each spray run had to be *personally* approved by President Kennedy. Not yet militarily committed, the US backed the southern Government's efforts from afar as they battled the North Vietnam Army (NVA) at the border, as well as the south Vietnamese insurgents closer to home, who fought for a unified Vietnam under Communist rule. These were the so-called Việt Cộng guerrilla fighters, often indistinguishable from rural civilians in the arable, and sometimes jungle, environment.

Success in Vietnam was deemed politically critical to Kennedy's term in office. Domestically there was growing racial tension: the Civil Rights movement had new figureheads demanding change while the Southern Manifesto, and those intent on upholding Jim Crow laws, were positioning themselves for a showdown. Both on land and in space, the U.S. found itself falling short of their Soviet counterparts. Sputnik 1 had given the Russians a lead in the Space Race in the late 50s and astronaut Yuri Gagarin had completed the first ever manned moon orbit in 1961. After the failed invasion of the Bay of Pigs (1961) and the Cuban Missile Crisis (1961), JFK spoke to a journalist of *The New York Times* immediately after his Vienna summit meeting with Soviet Premier Khrushchev, explaining, "now we have a problem making our power credible and Vietnam looks like the place."

Kennedy was not joking. He provided significant consultancy support to the Southern Government, led by President Ngô Đình Diệm, despite accusations of widespread brutality to his own people including the persecution of Buddhists. The now iconic photograph of the self-immolation of Buddhist monk, Thích Quảng Đức at a road intersection in Saigon, is probably the most famous protest against the alleged oppression. A man, engulfed in flames of his own making, committing to the ultimate sacrifice for his beliefs. Later that same year both Presidents, Diệm and Kennedy, were assassinated. It's almost impossible to determine if history may have taken alternative paths if JFK had continued in power but his presidential successor, Lyndon B. Johnson, ramped up involvement even further. After two alleged attacks on U.S. Navy ships in the Bay of Tonkin (alleged because subsequent intelligence suggests these were fabricated as a catalyst to declare war), the U.S. officially landed the first U.S. Marines in-country in March 1965.

"Only YOU can prevent a forest"

Grasping a metal shovel tightly in his left hand, his faded denim jeans belted up and sporting a yellow Forest Ranger campaign fedora, Smokey points directly at you from the poster, wide-eyed and expectant, requesting your help. Based on the famously impactful war recruitment propaganda, featuring Uncle Sam in the U.S. and Lord Kitchener in Britain, this illustrated American black bear works tirelessly on behalf of the U.S. Forest Service, championing the reduction of woodland fires in his native home. Frankly, he's sick of the alternative. Nearly nine out of every 10 wildfires in the States are caused by humans so the senior ranks drafted in Smokey Bear to educate a nation. And youngsters loved him. Smokey Bear soared in popularity in the 1940s appearing on radio programs, in comic strips, cartoons and as merchandise. At one stage he was the second most recognised symbol in American culture, behind Santa Claus.

"Only YOU can prevent forest fires!", was Smokey's iconic slogan. He was a hit and, as the years progressed, the number of fires did reduce.

His famous forest ranger campaign hat took a slightly sinister slant, however, by the early 1960s when a U.S. pilot got creative with one of the posters at the training base, leaving it reading, "Only YOU can prevent a forest!" The tweaked catchphrase spread like, well, wildfire, until it became the unofficial motto of Operation Ranch Hand. From Langley Air Force base in Virginia to the Bien Hoa base in Vietnam, edited posters popped up on the walls of briefing and training rooms, inspiring all that caught sight of them to follow Smokey's reworked guide and remove the forests.

Agent Orange was the chemical concoction sprayed to 'prevent', or remove, these forests but wasn't just dropped from helicopters and aeroplanes in Vietnam. Navy troops took barrels of the stuff, identified by an orange ring of paint marking each drum, on riverboats where they'd manually spray the bushes by the river edge. The aim was to kill vegetation and cover, driving the guerrillas back by spraying throughout the Mekong Delta; the vast maze of rivers, swamps and islands, home to floating markets, Khmer pagodas and villages surrounded by rice paddies. Strategic orders on all waterways came from the then top Naval Commander in Vietnam, Vice Admiral Elmo "Bud" Zumwalt Jr.

An accomplished and heavily decorated officer, the Californian was climbing the ranks of the U.S. Navy and, at the age of 48, found himself responsible for a flotilla of Swift Boats patrolling the coasts, harbours, and rivers of Vietnam. Bud was a huge man in stature, well over six feet in height, and carried a stocky, intimidating frame; his untamed, bushy eyebrows dominated his face and their stray angles characterised a man who would commandingly deliver orders daily. There was a personal twist to this campaign too, for the Vice

Admiral, as among his Swift-boat commanders was his 22-year-old son, Elmo Russell Zumwalt III, who'd signed up for the opportunity to serve his country under the direction of his father.

To tackle their 'invisible enemy', a force known to attack as if from nowhere and then disappear back into the jungle, Vice Admiral Zumwalt instructed his troops to defoliate the vast waterway arteries at the heart of the enemy's strategy, increasing visibility and shifting the balance of power back to the U.S. and South Vietnam forces. In just shy of ten years, ending in 1971, the U.S. sprayed approximately 91 million litres of herbicide killing over 5.5 million acres of forest and crop land. That's more than the land mass of Israel and removed enough crops to feed a population of 600,000 people for an entire year. To visualise the liquid volume here, think 36 Olympic swimming pools. Or the same volume of liquid needed for every person in a city the size of Glasgow to have a bath.

As the war progressed, the Northern government in Hanoi voiced their outrage at the use of herbicides claiming they were causing children to be born with terrible deformities, animals and fish to die, and their populations to develop other illnesses. The U.S. strongly dismissed this as nothing more than Communist propaganda; after all, their scientists had been clear that they couldn't harm human or animal life. William Bundy, assistant U.S. Secretary of State for the Far East, was particularly forceful, claiming these herbicides should not be classified as chemical weapons as they were not designed to harm people, they just played a supportive role in the war.

Whether known or not, however, this was not the case.

Exposure to Agent Orange had a direct impact on health, causing sarcoma, leukaemia, lymphoma and a variety of cancers including the lungs, larynx, trachea and prostate. Agent Orange contained a dioxin, namely TCDD; the most toxic compound of its type and, as it turns out, a human carcinogen causing cancers and other life-limiting diseases. As the herbicide saturated the land, the water table and permeated through communities of Vietnam, it became responsible for causing birth defects and abnormalities for decades to come. Once exposed, the chemicals were inhaled, or ingested in contaminated food or drink, or absorbed through the skin. The toxin could even gain access through contact with the eyes.

Adults exposed to the dioxin have given birth to children with the most horrendous disabilities. You only need to Google 'The Children of Agent Orange' to see the impact this so-called harmless weed killer has caused; a man writhes on a mattress as his mother cleans his open mouth; his body contorts, limbs angling in every direction beyond his control; he has complete neurological function, totally aware of his circumstances, caged in a body poisoned from the moment of conception. A young girl, maybe seven years old, runs down the dusty street with friends, her arms have not grown beyond her elbows and her legs, significantly different in length from each other, collide with the ground completely out of unison. But she's got the hang of it by now. She's had no choice. Her face contorts making it impossible for others to determine her emotions, unable as she is to vary her expression. The dioxins created a 'Nation of Mutation'.

As an aside, and while chronicled *ad nauseam*, it's worth briefly mentioning the humanitarian impact of the Vietnam War. Lasting 19 years, over 2.7 million U.S. military personnel served in Vietnam with 58,141 killed. The civilian death toll was conservatively in the region of 2 million people, with 5.3 million injured and over 11,000 becoming refugees in their own country. And Agent Orange wasn't the only chemical at play: you may have heard of "napalm", a cocktail of plastic polystyrene, hydrocarbon benzene and gasoline. It forms a sticky gel substance that, on explosion, continues to burn as it attaches itself to people's skin, hair, and clothing, causing unimaginable pain, severe burns, unconsciousness, asphyxiation, and often death. It reaches temperatures of 800-1,200 degrees C (1,500-2,200 degrees F) and the U.S. dropped almost 400,000 tons of napalm bombs in the decade between 1963 and 1973. If you had all those napalm bombs balanced on an exceptionally large weighing scale, and the Empire State building on the other side, the bombs would drop. And that's precisely what they did. Of the Vietnamese people who were on the receiving end, 60% suffered fifth-degree burns (meaning that the burn went down to the bone). Even William Bundy, the most ardent of defenders, wrote years later, "…in a nutshell, my present feeling is that it was a tragedy waiting to happen, but one made much worse by countless errors along the way, in many of which I had a part."[liii]

Despite the unspeakable horrors they witnessed and inflicted, U.S. military veterans returning to home shores at the end of March 1973 faced a new type of trauma. There was no 'welcome home' parade awaiting the vets, partly as there had been no mass demobilisation of troops. It had almost been like a nightclub 'one in, one out' policy for a decade: as soon as one soldier stepped onto home soil another took their place. Mooted celebrations in private were the order of the day.

Public opinion had been split throughout the war and returning soldiers were spat at by their society; figuratively and literally. While there were no Government benefits for G.I.s (Ground Infantry), members of the public voiced their anger at the national shame brought about by U.S. atrocities abroad. Support from the State to integrate back into civilian life and employment was pretty much 'non-existent' and the private sector were known to avoid employing former military personnel.

A nation had turned its back on the war veterans and, as financial hardships and mental health challenges continued to thwart their lives, they started to get cancer.

As the post-war years progressed an unusually high proportion of veterans, exposed to Agent Orange, developed types of cancer, life limiting diseases, or their children were born with birth defects. The very same biological issues the North Vietnamese had claimed were evident among their civilians during the war was now being experienced by American soldiers back home.

One of those affected was Elmo Russell Zumwalt III – son of 'Bud', the Navy Vice-Admiral. He'd developed lymphoma, then Hodgkin's disease, and subsequently his son, Russell, was born with severe learning disabilities.

Aptly named Elmo, after the patron saint of the sea, the elder Zumwalt had, by 1970, been promoted to Chief of Naval Operations, the top job, and set about bringing major reform to his area of the military. Fundamentally, in the wake of the Vietnam war, no civilians wanted to join the Navy. Difficulties recruiting and retaining naval personnel prompted Zumwalt to launch a series of policy directives known widely as 'Z-grams'. He started nice and easy by permitting beards and long hair followed by introducing beer-dispensing machines in the barracks. Then he really set to work. The treatment of minorities and women in the Navy was his specific concern, claiming regretfully that "racism and sexism were still an integral part of Navy tradition"[liv]. In his three years as Chief of Naval Operations (CNO), before retiring in 1973, he issued 121 Z-grams. Zumwalt's directives had tangible impact and formed foundational imperatives for reform in the Navy for decades to come.

This all led to Bud's face adorning the cover of Time Magazine in December of 1970 with the title, "The Military Goes Mod". An artistic portrait, with grey whisps now in his hair, a chiselled jawline and suitably depicted wild eyebrows, rests above a huge letter 'Z', filled with a diverse group of Navy personnel hard at work.

His focus in post-military years, however, was never far from his actions in Vietnam and accountability for ordering the mass usage of Agent Orange. As more cases surfaced, and it hit close to home, Bud was convinced that the herbicide he'd been charged with spraying on the Mekong Delta was directly responsible for causing his son's cancer, his grandson's learning disability, and the sickness and death of tens of thousands of other individuals (Chou, 2017). He decided he needed to do something to rebalance the scales.

Trying to right the wrongs

On the Western edge of the city of Milwaukee, Wisconsin, is the vast general hospital complex, neighbouring the city zoo, that houses one of the leading Medical Colleges in the State. Birthplace of the first self-contained underwater breathing apparatus (SCUBA) devices used by deep-sea divers, and the first to document Lyme Disease in a patient and pioneer treatment, it had long since been a magnet for original thinkers.

In the early 1970s a team of scientists at the Medical Centre had pioneered a forward-thinking practice of collaboration. A few years earlier the first successful hematopoietic cell transplantation (HCT) had taken place at the centre and researchers had a theory that if they could record the outcomes of transplantations in centres across the country they'd have a strengthened understanding of what types of treatment led to better outcomes. Sounds straightforward, right? Well, it was, but at the time this sort of openness was somewhat unique in medical practice, where even scientists on the opposite side of the same corridor, in differing areas of research, had no idea what their colleagues were working on. Then consider that this team were proposing to collect outcome data from centres in other cities and states nationwide.

In order for the intended project to work the key would be data capture; curating and analysing transplantation outcomes from medical centres across the U.S. The art of interrogating large data sets was perhaps quite new to medicine in the 1970s but had already demonstrated its merit in other fields for decades. Ironically, perhaps, nowhere more crucially than at sea through the documentation of tides, as we saw with Captain James Cook and the subsequent years of tidal discovery.

As someone that instinctively measured in 'knots' and 'kelvin', this unique approach the Milwaukee medical centre were taking in capturing best outcome data from bone marrow transplantations seized the attention of Admiral Elmo Zumwalt.

After staying the night at a hotel by the waterfront on Lake Michigan, the now retired Navy Admiral Zumwalt walked into the College grounds the next morning. His meeting with Mary Horowitz and Mortimer Bortin, leading medical figures developing pioneering outcomes data, was firmly with a view to finalise plans for a groundbreaking project. Bud had been using his significant platform to lobby for this project to receive Government funding in the highest corridors of power. "It is the first thing I think of when I awake in the morning', he explained to U.S. Congress, "and the last thing I remember when I go to sleep." He spoke of his actions in Vietnam, the spreading of deadly Agent Orange, and the life-limiting condition facing so many ex-service personnel – including his own son.

He also spoke of other successful registries around the world. Of emulating similar life-saving catalogues, and combining with industry-leading data analysis, to give hope and life to so many stricken with blood cancer. The campaign now had a very powerful, albeit unexpected, advocate[lv].

*

In 1986, in partnership with leading physicians and the ever-committed advocate, Bob Graves (Laura's father), Elmo Zumwalt and the U.S. Navy established the National Bone Marrow Donor Registry with one full-time employee housed at a tiny office in St. Paul, MN.

From the outset it was a partnership between the American Red Cross and the University of Minnesota providing computer support and data management. Working closely with Bob, and the Graves family, it got off to a fast start and in the first year, over 10,000 people signed up from across America. The registry performed their first donor search in September 1987 and, demonstrating immediately the national potential, a transplant took place in December that year where Diane Walters of Wisconsin donated marrow to 6-year-old Brooke Ward of North Carolina.

Over the subsequent years the registry grew in number and success. The founders knew the critical nature of collecting outcomes data and conducting collaborative research to improve results. The more names and results were added, the greater the probability of survival for someone faced with a life-limiting blood disease.

In its infancy, the project was unable to save the lives of Admiral Zumwalt's son or Laura Graves but has gone on to perform over 100,000 stem cell transplantations. Renamed 'Be The Match', it now acts as the global data hub with over 100 million Americans registered to donate.

Mind the gap
1993

Applause became ever more muffled in the background as Beverley, desperate to flee the stuffy, darkened labyrinth of tunnels clasped downward on the metal bar, unlocking her clunky escape to the icy chill of the night. She gasped at the air; hands on hips, neck tilted to the sky, it felt like the first actual breath she'd taken in hours. Her heart thumped in her ears. People bustled around but Beverley couldn't hear anything. She remembered nothing of the last claustrophobic ten-minutes, and she cared not to try, but in the unrestricted freedom of the city, a new anxiety opened its arms to her arrival.

Standing side of stage Beverley had waited, simply petrified. Pausing in the unlit wings she was invisible to the sell-out audience, crammed in over four floors. From her vantage, as the houselights rose, she could see them all, the whites of their eyes visible, their expressions now clear. Her stare darted around the auditorium, the luscious reds and golds adorning the theatre seeped into view, comforting grandeur with a distinct smell of fusty familiarity. The historic playhouse in East London looked majestic but this only added to the heightening pressure and expectation.

Dry night air chilled the sweat on her forehead as a man, she was unsure who, placed a hot chocolate carefully into her hands. She'd never spoken in front of so many people before. Something like 1,000 looking up and down at her, from the stalls to the rafters, as she told her story. At least she hopes she spoke the correct words, there is no way to know for sure. "Please do not leave here thinking 'how sad' and 'it is not my problem', Beverley had said. 'You *can* help. By becoming a donor and educating family and friends. No other community can help us." They seemed to listen, that had been her biggest fear. Being ushered on stage by the cast of the show, introduced by the acclaimed director whose performance had just finished entertaining a packed Hackney Empire, she'd feared more than anything that the crowd would grab their things and leave. OK, that would have been a blow for her own self-esteem, no doubt. But it was her son she worried for more. How would her eight-year-old cope if there was a mass exodus as his mum stood alone, almost begging these people for their help? Sat patiently in a cushioned red seat on the edge of an aisle, way past his bedtime and a little nonplussed by the performance he'd had to sit through, she feared such a dismissal would crush the hopes he'd placed in his community.

Sipping carefully from the steaming cardboard cup, she spotted him, her young Daniel, now sat ahead on the steps of a bus, parked in the road outside the venue. Despite the distance between them she saw his trademark smile, the same as it always was; broad, compelling and pure. With her partner Orin by his side, as he was inextricably by her own, Daniel jovially chatted and laughed with the volunteers that were operating the mobile health unit that night. And they waited. It could only have been minutes since she stepped off the stage - albeit it felt so much longer - and the main exits would soon be bustling, crowds navigating their ways home on night buses that trawled the capital's streets after hours, scooping and distributing their patrons from place to place.

Beverley's hope was, however, that people wouldn't go home with such haste. That they would stop off spontaneously at the health bus, take a blood test, and sign themselves onto a register. A register where their names may never even be called out but, if they ever were, they could save a person's life.

A frenzied spill onto the concourse. Hats and coats adorned to brace for the nip, a momentary freezeframe to collect their bearings. And then a stride to the bus. Not the one that takes them home, but the blood bus. A stream of souls ready to be tested, to leave their details, to try and save a life. To save her son's life. Beverley stood and welcomed as one-by-one, men and women shook her hand, offered their backing and rolled up their sleeves as a needle sucked in a liquid formula that could, perhaps, keep her Daniel alive.

Observing the queue, Beverley was awestruck. That they were overcoming their fears, the uncertainties and rumours, was inspiring. She wanted to hug them all. There were so many reasons why this was an important moment, many reasons why this was just the beginning, and a forward motion to make any significant difference to a wildly deficient circumstance. But observing the rows of Londoners standing in-line that evening to offer their DNA, Beverley knew this was a pivotal moment.

Daniel De-Gale had been diagnosed with acute lymphoblastic leukaemia (ALL) at the age of six and, like many others before him, needed a bone marrow donation if he had any chance of surviving. Customarily, his family were all tested – they'd have given every drop of blood had it ensured his life - including his younger sister Dominique, but with no success. It meant that he'd need a stranger, with a close to identical tissue type, to make a donation of their own stem cells.

His mother Beverley watched wearily as the last of the line-up gave their blood samples, the volunteers packaged and documented the process, and the concourse – recently a festival of noise and colour – quietened to a whisper. It was close to 2am. Daniel was asleep, carried in Orin's arms toward the car. As she set off to follow, thanking anyone she encountered on the way, she considered what difference the night could make. The doctors had explained Daniel's chances of finding a match. A probability to the tune of 1 in 250,000. The same as being struck and killed by a falling meteor. The queue of people had been long, but not that long. How many more of these events must she organise for her son to have any chance of finding that one?

She reached the car, still elated but cautiously understated. It had been over 20-years since experts performed the first unrelated bone marrow transplantation on a young boy in the same city. And he was still alive. Just above the River Thames in Westminster, perhaps less than 10-miles south, Simon Bostic had shown it was possible. So why, in 1996, were Beverley and Orin dragging their terribly sick son into the icy winter night to find that one needle in a haystack? The answer was linked to a vast blending of genes, historic experimentation, mistrust and abuse, and an underinvestment in inclusive progress. In short: it was because Daniel was Black.

In migration we trust

Dispersing from the theatre that night people travelled home to all corners of London. Catching buses, riding trains, hailing cabs and moving on foot: to Brixton, Peckham and Croydon in the south, Earls Court and Hammersmith way out west, and locally in Dalston, Haringey and Stratford in the east. Observed from a birds-eye view over the city, with the Hackney Empire as epicentre, a spread of travellers scattering hastily homeward, distributing in a seemingly random mosaic forged along well-trodden paths.

We've moved around as humans ever since we realised it was an option. Perhaps out of curiosity but more likely out of a desire to cultivate and thrive. Whatever the unknowns, one certainty is that it all began in Africa around 200,000 years ago.

Everyone living today that has non-African ancestors are descendants of the first travellers to leave that continent around 50,000 years ago. Those original pioneers migrated north and eastward, braving an untrodden route up over the treacherous mountainous passes into Asia – modern day Yemen, Saudi Arabia and Jordan. As the climate became dryer, and the Sahara Desert expanded, these explorers had no way of turning back so continued east, following a coastal route reaching modern-day Malaysia within a few millennia. It wasn't a race, there was no end destination in mind. These travellers and settlers, descendants of the first humans to leave Africa, were finding new ways to live in new environments. After 5,000 years of migration, sometime around 45,000 years ago, they reached Australia. We actually have no idea how they made the 90km ocean journey from what is now Indonesia – maybe by building rafts or fashioning floating devices like tree trunks – but we do know they landed on the island successfully.

At around the same time we find the first evidence of humans reaching Europe, too. A significantly shorter journey than Australia but challenging in a different way, with a harsh cold climate slowing any northerly progress. It's here that the first modern humans encountered their predecessors, the Neanderthals. To succeed in their travels and settlements, these humans had developed new skills including the use of tools, weapons and basic language – ingenuity which could have immediately led to the demise of the Neanderthal. But that would not occur for another few thousand years – the two living alongside one another in relative harmony, interbreeding and coexisting across Southern Europe until the Neanderthals died out around 40,000 years ago.

Then came the most recent ice age, sometime around 15,000 years ago, transforming much of the earth's surface into an inhospitable freeze. Across many lands new barriers of glacier separated groups of people while in others sea levels dropped so dramatically that lands, once oceans apart, became connected. This saw the first migration of humans to today's North America navigating a 'bridge' that rose between Siberia and Alaska – a strip of land where the Bering Strait exists today. From this point they slowly travelled south and these first settlers are the ancestors of today's native Americans. It's quite something that by this point in history, around 10,000 years ago, humans had managed to inhabit every continent on earth – except Antarctica – having started a relatively short time before from a small corner of Africa. Once settled, languages began to form, unique based on their surroundings and interactions; all precursors of the way we communicate with one another today. Scattered around the world these small populations of people gradually became increasingly distinct from one another linguistically, culturally and genetically.

Every single member of a species is unique. We may resemble our parents, our siblings or other relatives, but each of us has distinctive characteristics that make us who we are. It's Rosalind Franklin's discovery, DNA, that is unique; that code is what determines traits like our hair colour, skin colour, personality. All this data is stored in four types of *nitrogenous base*, namely: adenine (A), cytosine (C), guanine (G) and thymine (T). They pair up along the twisted ladder and each human cell contains around 3 billion pairs. You can think of it like combinations of letters filling the pages of this book. The pairs can be ordered in many different sequences forming the genes. The complete sequence of DNA of a species, when the book is finished, is the genome[30].

Due to the mass migrations and distinct populations mixing, the diversity of DNA sequences has increased over time. Known as 'recombination', or mating, it has led to the human genome becoming more varied with lots of little differences. As these blended characteristics survive natural selection – overcoming the challenge of predators, climate, disease, and others – they pass on robust attributes in mixed code to their offspring, further changing the gene pool and expanding the makeup of a species. When you consider that 99% of all species ever to have existed on earth are now extinct, the way humans have evolved is a sure sign of success. One such adaptation we've made for survival is a very visually obvious one, our skin colour. Melanin is a superb natural sunscreen. This polymer has been present for billions of years, seen in our earliest ancestors, to protect us against ultraviolet radiation from the sun. Our bodies need that radiation, specifically UVB rays, which we use to create Vitamin D – a key tool used to absorb calcium, strengthening our bones. But too much UVB rays is not good news: this radiation can damage skin cells, produce sunburn and is thought to cause most skin cancers. This is where melanin comes into play. It forms an ultraviolet shield from the powerful glare. For humans living closer to the Equator – Earth's closest point to the sun – more melanin protection means darker skin pigmentation and a stronger shield. Nature working at its best.

Given our starting point in Africa, the skin of the earliest members of our lineage, namely *Homo erectus* around 1.8-million years ago, was darkly pigmented. That heritage is true for every living human on

---

[30] Explanation given at the Future of Tomorrow museum exhibit, Rio de Janeiro, November 2022

earth today. But as our ancestors migrated across the globe to new climates, further away from the Equator, they were less exposed to ultraviolet from the sun. They needed to weaken the shield a little to let some more UVB rays through for Vitamin D production. So, our skin began to adapt, changing colour to fit with the surroundings. The darkly pigmented peoples would be found along the line of the Equator and, the further north and south you travelled from that line, the lighter the skin progressively became.

These changes took place over tens of thousands of years as our species evolved to survive in our newfound habitats. As population groups grew, moved and mixed over these many millennia, evolutionary diversity increased.

With the ice age behind them, and the climate enjoying greater sunshine and rainfall, crops and animals were in plentiful supply, encouraging populations to settle in one place. Fertility of the soil, and of the populous, enabled a pivotal moment, the effects of which significantly influence how we live today. A new concept, agriculture, thrived the world over in places where humans lived and this comfortable and plentiful new lifestyle led to a surge in family sizes. This, in turn, reduced the appeal in nomadism favouring instead the desire to put down roots – figuratively and literally. Population groups thrived in pockets across the map. While static for some time, our ancestors would start to travel again as invention led to improved transportation and they once again set out to acquire land, jobs and trade goods. At this point they encountered other large groups – quite similar to themselves, yet markedly different – and new families created in these 'meetings' of distant cultures fused genetic characteristics further.

Other mass migrations from Africa have taken place in more recent history, but these were not self-determined. In roughly 360 years, between 1500 and the 1860s, approximately 12-million African people were forcibly taken to the Americas in the largest involuntary relocation in history. A scattering of millions consisting of some 50 ethnic and linguistic groups were enslaved in North America, South America and the Caribbean – as well as in Europe. These abhorrent relocations, and eventual emancipations, transformed the diversity of countries; not just phenotypically - observable physical characteristics, such as hair type, eye pigmentation, skin colour - but new meetings of unique groups led to further blend distinct genomes.

All this goes to show that, no matter how different we look from the person opposite us on the bus or someone we see on TV from a country far away, we're all fundamentally share the same back story. Equally, however, differences that *do* exist are not skin deep; they go much further than that.

We're all different

Variations in genetic characteristics are best thought of more in terms of probabilities than rigid demarcations[31]. Put simply: to be tall in stature with blonde hair may be common among those from Nordic countries but not all Nordics are tall with blonde hair, nor are all owners of height and fairer follicles indeed of Nordic descent. When the species began there were thousands of possible genetic variations and, as we've migrated and mixed over the millennia, these have mutated and multiplied. Our DNA similarities have become less and less making each distinct group of people less and less consanguineous (the percentage of genetic similarities two

---

[31] Steven Marsh article, Anthony Nolan charity: Race and genetics in stem cell transplantation - BioNews

people have). As we've seen in transplantation, the closer the characteristics, or consanguinity, between the donor and recipient the better the chance that the transplant will 'take' or succeed. Again, it all comes down to Human Leukocyte Antigen (HLA) type – the human *Major Histocompatibility Complex (MHC)* – and our ability to confuse the proteins in our immune system to determine between the self and the non-self.

Over time distinct HLA types have developed through migrations and mutations across the globe. For example, an Australian Aboriginal tissue type is markedly different from a white northern European which again is distinctly different from someone living in the favellas of Rio de Janeiro or the bustling suburbs of Mumbai. If you have mixed heritage, perhaps you are African-Caribbean British like Daniel De Gale, this gets somewhat more complicated. It is probable that your distinct HLA type will come from a mix of African origins, with perhaps some native South American genes and maybe some white northern European ancestry. For an individual with this breadth of diversity in their genes, they would need a donor with similar diversity.

For a Caucasian Brit, the same age and with the same diagnosis as Daniel, their chances at the time were around 20% at best of finding a matching donor. For Daniel, and many other Black British people in the same circumstance, that probability was around 0.0004%.

This situation wasn't only down to diverse genotypes, however, albeit that was, and remains, a significant challenge. What Beverley and Orin discovered as they navigated this complicated new nightmare, was a staggering indifference and dismissiveness among the Black African-Caribbean community when it came to becoming potential stem cell donors.

Fear and encoding

It was April 1973 that the first unrelated bone marrow transplant took place with Simon Bostic and, as we know, many more soon followed in Seattle and other institutions around the world. So why are we focusing on Daniel's story which took place almost three-decades later. When donor registers brimmed with stem cell options - from a basement broom cupboard in London, to the Navy backed campaign in the States - hundreds of thousands put themselves forward to see if their graft could make a difference. Through the years, however, the register saw an ever-expanding melanin gap on both sides of the Atlantic; empty spaces in the list where potential donors from the African, Caribbean and Mixed Heritage community should have been.

The prospect of giving away something from inside your body can, to many, seem quite daunting. And with good reason. If it's functioning, then surely you need it. Disinterest in and suspicion of bone marrow donation – or any blood or organ donation for that matter – was particularly prevalent within the African-Caribbean community. We continue to see hesitation to this day, be it elective uptake of routine scans, vaccinations or screenings, certain groups of the population remain underrepresented due to personal choice. Since its inception myth, rumour and fear has cloaked stem cell treatment. So, what are the barriers, some perceived and others very real, when it comes to mass engagement with medicine?

First and foremost, the extraction of stem cells is often referred to as 'harvesting' which comes with its own connotations of plucking crops in their prime. The cells are located in a spongy substance deep in the core of your larger bones - the reason extraction often happens in the hip bone - access to which is achieved by inserting a needle. Not such an appealing prospect, even if you're OK with needles, and this was regularly the most common fear cited by prospective donors. Immediately followed by 'does it hurt?' Of course, when this treatment first began the needles were long and intimidating, the pain relief was less effective and tales of the process, well documented and long-lasting in the collective memory, were somewhat traumatic. More recently it is less off-putting, carried out with precise equipment under general anaesthetic in an operating room using sterile techniques – but some legends take time to die out.

Another fear often cited, as with many similar procedures, are the possible side effects experienced by the donor. By giving away your body's cells will you leave yourself vulnerable? During the procedure, you will be relieved of approximately two litres of bone marrow. Yes, this may seem like a large amount, but it represents less than 10% of your stem cells. It may help to know that your body makes more than 200-billion blood cells in your bone marrow every day. Your cell supply is usually topped up and back to normal levels within four to six weeks, though your body can function perfectly fine in the meantime.

But fears don't arise from nowhere. In fact, when staff nurse Frances Otto-Depner provided her stem cells to Laura Graves in the Fred Hutchinson, she went on to have a long series of health complications as a direct result of her donation. She remained resolute that she had no regrets despite the patient eventually not surviving and her own life being impacted hugely. Today just around 2.4% of donors experience a serious complication.

But for many years there was one question above all others asked by those cautious of donating their bone marrow: *"What if they can clone me?"* Of course, while their motive to do so is unconvincing, the answer had very recently been proved to be, *'yes, they probably can'*. Just months before Beverley stepped out onto the stage in Hackney, the world was introduced to Dolly; a female sheep born in Midlothian, Scotland, and the first mammal cloned from an adult somatic cell. Dolly was the starting point and clones of monkeys, pigs, deer, horses and bulls followed. While contentious, researchers now see cloning as a potential way to preserve endangered species.

But whatever a person's reasons for not joining the register, no matter how genuine or trivial, surely that is their decision to make? Even if it were to likely save a life; should that resolution not still be your personal choice? These cells *belong* to you; surely no one can force you?

In the United States in 1978, former Pennsylvania asbestos worker Robert McFall developed a rare disease called aplastic anaemia; his blood had stopped producing the required armour to battle infection. He desperately needed a bone marrow transplant from a matching donor. After a narrow search his first cousin, David, was found to be the only possible match however, when asked if he'd donate his bone marrow, David politely declined.

Robert, desperate to live, did what anyone else would do in his situation. He sued his cousin. OK, perhaps not everyone would do that, but the case appeared in county court where the ruling was made quickly in favour of David. While stating a refusal to offer bone marrow was "morally indefensible", Judge Flaherty refused to force the cousin to donate his stem cells as this "would impose a rule which would know no limits, and one could not imagine where the line would be drawn".

It goes right back to the Fourth Amendment of the United States Constitution in 1792, "The right of the people to be secure in their persons...", a recognition of the universal and fundamental natural right of bodily integrity.

A long-standing fundamental right for all Americans… unless you were Black.

All just a little bit of history repeating

Trepidation, suspicion and mistrust among Black people is often rooted in historic events, exacerbated by recent and current health inequalities. Its aetiology is often recognised as the Tuskegee syphilis study, starting in 1932, where the purpose was to observe untreated syphilis in African American men. The United States Public Health Service (PHS) and the Centers for Disease Control and Prevention (CDC) lied to the men, telling them they were receiving free healthcare for their participation; they were not. They were simply being observed. Government and medical leaders watched as this completely treatable disease killed over 100 African American men, infected 40 of the patients' wives, and 19 children were born with congenital syphilis. This ethically abusive study was due to last for six-months yet only concluded in 1972, 40-years later.

Fear of medicine, caused by unwilling participation of Black people in experiments of torture, abuse, and humiliation at the hands of doctors has been described as Black iatrophobia by writer Harriet A. Washington. For more than four centuries, Washington states, there has been a biomedical enterprise designed to exploit African-Americans which is a principal contributor to current mistrust.[lvi]

Persistent attitudinal divides may be strongly influenced by sustained racial disparities in health, limited access to health care, and negative encounters with health care providers. It may also be due to individual stories – those occasional benchmark cases - where medical injustice was inflicted on Black people. Cases such as that of Henrietta Lacks. You may be aware of Henrietta's story – a best-selling book and movie[lvii] have brought it to a global audience – but the unethical practice of another highly esteemed academic institution is worth mentioning.

There was a rumour when growing up on the streets of Baltimore. If children misbehaved their parents would tell them they'd be snatched straight from the streets by the mad scientists at Johns Hopkins University for medical experiments. It was a little dramatic - intended to correct behaviour - but turned out to be quite close to the bone.

On 29th January 1951, Henrietta walked into Johns Hopkins suffering from an acute pain in her womb. At the time, this was the only local hospital that would treat Black patients and, after a biopsy was taken, she was soon diagnosed with cervical cancer. Treatment started straight away but, without Henrietta's knowledge or consent, two samples were taken from her cervix – one healthy, the other cancerous - and handed to cell biologist, George Gey.

As unsettling and unethical as this may appear, that a part of your body can be taken from you entirely without you knowing, it's something that could happen to any of us. To this day, patient consent is not required for research on human tissue obtained during medical treatment, but only on one condition; that the 'donors" identity is removed.

When observing Lacks' cancerous cells, Gey noticed that they reproduced at an incredibly high rate, staying 'alive' much longer than any other cells they'd worked with once out of the body. In fact, they were doubling in number every 24-hours allowing Gey and his team so much more scope to experiment. Meanwhile Henrietta's ongoing treatment didn't seem to be making much difference and the cancer metastasised throughout her body. On 4th October 1951, 31-year-old Henrietta died at Johns Hopkins. Realising the unique characteristics of Henrietta's cells, Gey wasted no time and ordered an assistant to extract more cell samples from her dead body while it lay waiting for autopsy. To remove the patient's identity, Gey used a simple method of taking the first two letters from a first and last name. These cells would forever be known as HeLa.

Over the next 70+ years – now distributed extensively to scientists around the world - Henrietta's cancer cells continued to replicate quickly and aggressively. Due to their unique characteristics, they have been at the root of some of the most seismic developments in medical science. They were used to develop the polio vaccine, sent into Space to experiment at zero gravity, influenced AIDS and chemotherapy treatment, In vitro fertilization (IVF) and even the vaccine for cervical cancer. More recently scientists worked with HeLa cells to better understand the infectivity of SARS-CoV-2 (COVID-19). There's unlikely to be a person on earth today that has not, in some way, benefitted from Henrietta's cells.

HeLa cells were the first human cells to be successfully cloned, just four years after Henrietta's death in 1955. There are over 11,000 registered patents involving HeLa cells[lviii]. And they simply keep on replicating, seemingly never ending. HeLa cells became the first 'immortal' human cell line to reproduce infinitely in a lab and have been replicated so prolifically that laid end-to-end they could be wrapped around the earth three times[32].

And yet, while Henrietta's cells can be defined as one of the greatest medical contributions of all time, Henrietta did not knowingly contribute them. Nor, too, were her close family – mourning their loved one – made aware that her cells were being farmed out across the planet. In fact, her family were subjected to further unethical trials. Under the guise of checking that they too didn't suffer from the same cancerous disease, they were in fact unknowingly 'donating' their blood so it could be genetically tested for the same

---

[32] HeLa cells (1951) | British Society for Immunology

unique traits.

This could, and probably did, happen with other people through medical history and, while skin colour may not have defined ethical decisions, it's yet another reason why African American and African Caribbean families became increasingly sceptical about medicine.

Finally bridging the gap

When lists of names flourished, each clunkily clicked into the bone marrow register held on early Personal Computers (PCs) in the mid-1980s, it would have been easy to miss what was hidden in plain sight. Very few of the names being input belonged to those of African American or African Caribbean heritage. The mistreatment and ethical crimes of the past now further victimised Black people who, in need of a donor or potentially life-saving treatment, would avoid the halls of medical institutions as stories they heard as children still echoed in their ears.

Fear passed down in the fabric of a family. If not explicitly told, implicitly inferred. They could feel it in their bones. For a Black child in Britain, like Daniel De Gale, it was the inside of their bones that he needed them to share.

Daniel sat up in his hospital bed at Great Ormond Street Hospital, in London, on high alert. His palms were sweating and Orin, sat in the chair alongside him, grabbed his hand tightly. He sensed his son's tension. But he never gave up hoping.

Can they score? They always score.

Daniel's transplant had been due to take place a few days before but there were complications and a delay. That didn't concern Daniel. His oversized replica shirt drowned the Manchester United fan as he longed for his side to find something, anything, to save this match. It was the Champions League Final, 26th May 1999; the pinnacle of European club football and his heroes were moments away from defeat against Bayern Munich, of Germany.

He prayed someone rescue the match. His parents prayed a match could rescue him.

As Teddy Sheringham and Ole Gunnar Solskjær scored dramatic late goals, crowning Daniel's team as champions, his dad Orin inwardly revelled in the fact the transplant had been delayed. They'd waited for so long, and were desperately running out of time, but to see his boy jumping around his bed, jubilant and singing wearing the famous red and white, was an observed moment he knew he'd treasure. Orin cried tears of happiness at the result; not for the team – he supported Chelsea – but he knew Daniel could never have enjoyed this thrill during recovery from a transplant. The postponement was a beautiful blessing in disguise.

A few weeks later, on the 16th June 1999, 12-year-old Daniel's bone marrow transplant took place at Great Ormond Street Hospital. Stem cells that approximately matched his own had been tracked down in Detroit, Michigan, thanks to the Anthony Nolan register and the partner American Bone Marrow Register. Sat on a bed, still proudly wearing his oversized football jersey, a *Hickman Line* catheter tube fed new stem cells, belonging to donor Doreene Carney, into his weakened body. Daniel became the first Black person to receive an unrelated bone marrow transplant in the UK.

Beverley and Orin were over-the-moon, and they were not finished. When they first heard Daniel's diagnosis, less than 0.2% of donors on the register were from African communities. A staggeringly low percentage. It needed redressing. The Anthony Nolan Trust worked closely to support their efforts, including volunteering on the bus outside the Hackney Empire that night, but they simply didn't have the database to work with. Then Daniel's story stirred something. Beverley and Orin established a group called the African-Caribbean

Leukaemia Trust (ACLT) before the transplant to help raise awareness in London and beyond. Families signed up, donations started to be made, awareness began to grow. This had become something bigger. What if their passion could now go on to save the lives of people from African-Caribbean communities in the UK?

It was a full 26 years after Simon Bostic's unrelated transplant; 25 years since the bone marrow register was formally established just down the road in Westminster, only a few miles from where Daniel's transplant finally took place. In that quarter of a century, not a single Black person in the UK had received a successful unrelated donation due to the lack of suitable matches in what was now a global network of registers operating in countries around the world. The de Gale's, through ACLT and a collection of sporting and celebrity ambassadors, were intent on changing this narrative for Black communities, with or without the support of those in positions of political power. They started the vital work to actively redress the melanin imbalance, a final piece in the puzzle of a volunteer registry, initiated 26-years prior by Liz Bostic. To truly make Liz and Shirley's concept of a donor registry a success, it needed to be accessible by all people equally.

What happened next?

On 8th October 2008, the same day that Françoise Barré-Sinoussi and Luc Montagnier were presented with their Nobel Prize for the discovery of HIV, 21-year-old Daniel De Gale died of multiple organ failure. A little over eight-years earlier he had become the first Black person in the UK to receive a stem cell transplant from an unrelated volunteer donor and, while granting him extra years of life, it sadly didn't offer a full recovery. The extra years were due to collaboration between global bone marrow registers, kick-started in London in 1974, and his unrelated donor was found in Detroit, Michigan.

This solution was unthinkable in the 1960s. A child diagnosed with a blood disease would have had, at best, a 10% chance of surviving to adulthood. The unknowns were vast and progress slow. Trials mostly resulted in error; scores of children died painful deaths in the arms of desperate parents. The concept of globally searchable registers was science fiction.

By the end of the 1980s, the landscape had transformed. This 30-year period was, and remains, arguably the most transformational era in the history of blood disease. Filled with iconic parents, pioneering scientists and impactful mass media campaigning. Future research has achieved great things, such as cord blood transplants and next generation DNA sequencing, but none would have been conceived without progress during this significant stretch of time.

At the time of Daniel's acute lymphoblastic leukaemia (ALL) diagnosis in 1993, unrelated bone marrow donations had been taking place for 20 years since the very first transplant of Simon Bostic. Her Royal Highness, Princess Anne, opened a brand-new bone marrow unit at the Westminster Children's Hospital in June, 1985[lix] and, after many clinical successes of the 1970s and 80s, charities like Save the Children and health authorities started taking the treatment more seriously, investing significantly to resource experts with whatever they needed to save lives.

It's impossible to know if an earlier match would have changed the outcome for Daniel. What's undeniable, though, is that the ACLT (African-Caribbean Leukaemia Trust), established by his parents Beverley and Orin before his death, has gone on to save numerous lives through advocacy, changing policy, increasing diversity on the bone marrow registers and gifting possibility to people facing diagnosis today. The seeds sown all those years ago, and the subsequent numbers of donors now registered, has unequivocally proven their community has risen to the challenge. The work isn't complete, you probably still need a pool of 10-20 times more potential donors to find a match for a Black British patient, but now there are so many more names on the register to choose from.

Increasingly, volunteer registries across the world communicate, collaborate and exchange to find the best possible outcomes for patients.

Transatlantic blood donations, from the United States to Britain, started in 1940 when Charles Richard Drew led the Blood for Britain campaign during World War II. His pioneering work, optimising transfused plasma, led him to a job supplying blood to the U.S. Army and Navy with the American Red Cross in February 1941. It was a short-lived career move. Drew quit in 1942, protesting to the policy of separating the blood of African Americans from those of white donors. Himself an African American, his was a short-lived life, in general.

Drew, for many years, attended the annual free clinic at the John A. Andrew Memorial Hospital in Tuskegee, Alabama. It was a teaching hospital that provided postgraduate training to Black physicians and one of the only nearby hospitals that would treat Black patients. Unbeknownst to Drew, and colleagues, the infamous Tuskegee Syphilis Study was already underway within the very same building. Driving himself and three colleagues to the annual event from Washington, DC, in 1950, Drew lost control of his car near Burlington, North Carolina, somersaulting multiple times and landing in a field. He was taken to a nearby hospital but his injuries proved fatal, dying just 30-minutes after arrival. He was 45-years old. Rumours circulated that, in a cruel irony, the hospital had refused him a blood transfusion on account of not having enough beds for Black patients. It was a baseless claim; his colleague, a survivor of the accident, strongly refuted the rumour, expressing a view that Drew's injuries were so severe he'd never have survived. But his story added to myths around medical treatment for non-White people in America at this time.

When Dr David James diligently worked in the basement broom cupboard, he realised diversity of HLA was key to solving this riddle. After years of exploration, he and colleagues identified 26 different sub-types of Human Leucocyte Antigen (HLA); the unique barcode that differentiates every human on earth. Understanding this enigma within our blood, Dr David James was able to contribute to numerous world firsts, including the unrelated bone marrow transplant of Simon Bostic, along with twin, sibling and parent-child transplants.

Despite this, they'd not entirely cracked the code. Many patients continued to die without medical salvation with huge unknowns regarding the diversity of HLA proteins. They realised that the protein itself came in very many flavours. Working outwards from the family, each of us have 12 HLA proteins: six inherited from the father, six from the mother. Siblings, especially identical, are the most likely to have comparable HLA and the wider family members will have similarities, albeit less and less 'matching' the further removed they become.

The extent of diversity was not immediately apparent. In subsequent years, Dr James' analysis was developed further and soon it was realised how little they in fact knew during those early years. From their understanding of 26 sub-types of HLA, there are now known to be over 35,000 variations of the protein, and that number continues to grow the more that humans diverge and procreate.

Knowing the importance of diversified registers isn't the end of the challenge. In Brazil, for example, there exists one of the largest and most diverse human populations on the planet today. Over 214-million people are spread far and wide across the fifth largest country by landmass, their origins a mix of Indigenous, European, African and Asian, covering all corners of the 8.5-million square kilometres (just shy of a quarter of the Moon's surface area). Slavery and colonisation have shaped this diversity, as has the sheer size, accessibility and traditional rural communities that continue to exist and thrive in remote corners of the country (mostly in the northern Amazonian regions). A glorious mix that culturally adds so much to the country is somewhat more complicated when it comes to tackling blood disease.

REDOME (Registro Brasileiro de Doadores Voluntários de Medula Óssea) is the Brazilian volunteer bone marrow register, established by José Roberto Feresin de Moraes in São Paulo in 1993, tasked with matching stem cell demands domestically and internationally. It's a huge challenge which initially, like other registers around the world, began with no public funding and just a few resolute researchers. Finding a suitably close match, in a crowd so diverse and dispersed, is an ongoing challenge that lead coordinator, Dr Danielli Oliveira, and her team now based in Rio de Janeiro, are constantly looking to tackle.

Frenchman George Mathé continued to be all-or-nothing in his approach. Brilliantly innovative, equally chaotic and rarely able to bring many of his best ideas to fruition clinically. He was described by peers as stimulating but ineffectual. But he kicked things off in this story with his treatment of the nuclear scientists at Vinca. He demonstrated what *could* be possible.

Don Thomas, in Seattle, was somewhat different. More methodical, systematic and focused, he was better able to bring together a team of experts and keep them engaged to achieve meaningful impact. Don was never in the lab; he left the detailed investigations and clinical work to his team, while always ensuring his name appeared on all the research papers. It led to Don's award of the Nobel Prize in Medicine in 1990, taking Bob and Sherry Graves as his guests to the ceremony in Sweden. It was justified global recognition for a career focused on stem cell transplantation but not something his close colleagues at The Hutch ever achieved themselves. Those co-workers are not talked about today in the same breath as Don, something they explain isn't necessarily something they hold against him, but something not quickly forgotten.

Like so many examples in this book, a timely coming together of inquisitive scientists and inexplicably fortuitous events led to discoveries and treatments that saved countless lives.

That is not to say everything was rosy from then on.

Despite thousands of deaths, the AIDS epidemic only finally

engaged the American public's attention when Hollywood actor Rock Hudson announced his diagnosis in 1985. Michael Gottleib, the doctor that first raised the alarm about the autoimmune disease, was his personal physician but after months of hospital treatment in Paris and Los Angeles, Hudson died in October of that same year.

This was a landmark moment for AIDS. That a household name could die brought the news home to millions of Americans, and people worldwide, that had previously considered the disease inconsequential. Hudson had never disclosed his homosexuality, something that he felt may have negatively impacted his career, claiming instead that initial trips to the hospital were for treatment of liver cancer. Leading medical figures faced public derision for their work to tackle the 'gay disease'. Among them, Michael Gottleib and Joel Weisman, the two figures credited with discovering AIDS. The more openly they voiced their concerns, the more peers gave them the cold-shoulder professionally. Prominent institutions actively downplayed rumours that their corridors were places this troublesome disease was being treated. It was deemed "unbecoming" for academics to talk about it in the media (Kinsella, 1989). In fact, a few years after identifying AIDS, Gottleib claims his newfound fame may have led to his tenure being revoked by UCLA, forcing him into private practice despite being the first to document one of the deadliest diseases of the 20th century[lx].

As we now know, around 32.7 million people have died from AIDS-related illness since the beginning of the epidemic. In September 1985, the American Foundation for AIDS Research (amfAR) was formed. Dr. Michael Gottleib became its Founding Chair, and actor Elizabeth Taylor, its National Chair. One of its first donations was a gift of $250,000 from Rock Hudson shortly before he died.

Professor Rainer Storb, who established allogeneic stem cell transplantation at the Fred Hutch in Seattle, still works at the centre today, as Head of Transplantation Biology Program in the Clinical Research Division. He swapped commuting by bike to commuting by kayak, travelling Seattle's waterways, Lakes Washington and Union, still managing to dodge the traffic. As well as competitively rowing in his mid-80s, he continues to dedicate his career to eliminating the barriers to successful transplant, including GvHD, and has focused much of his work to lessening the toxicity of treatment for patients with leukaemia. His introduction of non-myeloablative transplantation, sometimes called a "mini-transplant," involves minimal pre-transplant radiation and has been particularly impactful at extending the lives of older patients.

Armand Keating, once a colleague of Storb in the early days of the Hutch, returned to his native Canada in 1982 and used his experience in Seattle to help co-found the volunteer bone marrow register there. Also Toronto-based is Jim Till, one-half of the team that identified and proved the functionality of the stem cell. His research over 70-years sees the biophysicist still active at the University of Toronto, now as Professor Emeritus, with recent years dedicated to promoting the importance of open access to scientific research. Like many other instances in this book, and throughout science, his fortunate discovery with Ernest McCulloch founded a base-level of cellular understanding from which much scientific and medical advancement flourished.

While fortunate moments occur all-the-time in medicine, the convergence of Liz and Shirley at that precise time wasn't serendipity: the latter actively travelling across the world to emulate the path of the former. The connection of these two incredibly passionate and unrelenting women played no small part in the outcomes we see today all these years on.

Shirley mused about ending it all, giving up in the face of an unforgiving nemesis, but Liz kept encouraging, making comparisons to her own experience. She ensured that Shirley continued fighting. Shirley added a section in her memoir about Liz, "someone who gave me the courage to fight on deserves a lasting memory"

Unlike Liz, the end of Shirley's life was very much intentional. A note she left displayed her intent, "I hope today I can end the horror my life has become." After years of living with Parkinson's disease she'd made her views on euthanasia extremely clear. She'd already tried to end her life once in an attempt she described as 'botched'.

She succeeded in taking her own life, aged 59, in December 2001. At the time of her death, 30,000 possible donors were registered to the registry and 2,300 had received life-saving transplants. For her relentless commitment to the bone marrow register, she received an Order of the British Empire (OBE) from The Queen for services to charity.

In a story about the life and influence of Liz Bostic, it could be tempting to ignore or supress the impact of another. To downplay another mother's achievements to favour the narrative. In this story, both Liz and Shirley played vital roles and benefitted enormously from each other.

By the time Liz and Shirley met, Simon's world-first transplant had already been completed and years of public campaigning had been front-page news in countries around the world. But without Shirley's fresh energy and structured vision, Liz's ideas and progress may have fizzled out in favour of a quiet and comfortable home life. More than fundraising for new isolation tents or additional nurse salaries, Shirley brought logistical solutions to Liz's problem. Similarly, and crucially, Shirley Nolan 'the campaigner', simply would not have existed without Liz Bostic. In her, Shirley saw what was possible, how far a mother's quest could take a family in search of salvation. Liz demonstrated how to use the media, how to navigate the corridors of power within medical research and inspired Shirley to move her family to the other side of the world to face this problem head on. They shared a steadfast resolve to take her message to anyone who would listen, and to shake up those who would not[lxi]. Without Liz Bostic, the bone marrow transplantation register would not have happened as it did.

It's easy to conclude that, in the fullness of time, the bone marrow register would inevitably been created. If not Liz Bostic and Shirley Nolan, or even Bob Graves, another parent of another dying child would have moved things forward, pushing the medical world and the public to invest in new solutions. Perhaps this is true, but a few things are worth remembering.

Firstly, while we can assume a registry was bound to happen at some point, the fact remains that it came about at this specific time and according to the details laid out in this book. Without rewriting history, or dwelling on conjecture, accumulated scientific understanding gathered over centuries led to this institution and individuals in central London making a monumental leap.

Secondly, the context of bone marrow transplantation at the time shows there was very little patience remaining. Inside and outside hospitals, this practice was all but discredited with decades of failure leaving observers aghast that it was still being trialled. A world-first and registry could have happened in the years following Liz and Shirley but, with lack of funding and too much failure overwhelming, it is possible the small teams would have been forced to down tools in the not-too-distant future. In short, the whole operation was close to being completely shut down.

Timing is everything. Perhaps this is why Simon Bostic's transplant was heralded a resounding triumph. That the world's first 'successful' unrelated bone marrow transplantation happened at this precise time. Jack Hobbs knew it was now or never for bone marrow transplantation and, come what may, this little boy would show the world that his work needed to be taken seriously.

It caused conflict. John Barrett, among others, felt the approach a little gung-ho and lacking scientific evidence to back it up. After all, soon after the transplant Simon's samples showed no donor blood in his system. His donor's stem cells had immediately gone to work, new personnel in the blood factory, producing lots of new white blood cells and sending them around the body. There just weren't enough of them. A few weeks in, his original stem cells overwhelmed the newer 12%, gradually but emphatically flushing them out. The physicians had feared this may happen, but they'd been terrified that grafting more ran the very real risk of deadly Graft vs Host Disease. Simon's body would simply have been too weak to recover.

What they did learn about is displacement. That if they replicated this procedure using only 12% on another patient, it would surely fail again.

Without Hobbs' best-foot-forward methodology, bone marrow transplantation could have failed too. More specifically, the register would almost certainly never have happened.

News of the transplant definitely wouldn't have reached Australia and, in turn, Shirley Nolan unquestionably wouldn't have brought Anthony to London. She wouldn't have campaigned for volunteer donors to register and a structured index would not have been fashioned at that time.

2023 marks 50-years since the world's first ever unrelated bone marrow transplant. That Friday 13th in April 1973 when three-year old Simon Bostic received donated stem cells at the Westminster Children's Hospital in Vincent Square, London.

Since that landmark day, Simon (or 'Lazarus', as his doctors since dubbed him) has lived a challenging yet vibrant life. His health has never been 100%, always an unwanted companion in a half-century packed with travel, celebration, learning and love. Despite medication and tubes following him wherever he goes, Simon has remained resolutely unwilling to allow any malfunctions to curtail zest for action. His travels have taken him deep into the Amazon rainforest, the mountains of Uganda, through the outback of Australia and, more recently, on safari in South Africa. He married Christopher, his long-term partner, in 2015 and they live overlooking the North Downs in Surrey.

In a quiet and personal ceremony in 2022, devised and officiated by a close friend and vicar, Simon finally had the opportunity to say goodbye to his mum and brother. Deprived of the chance to attend either funeral as a boy, we talked on one of our many meetings about the lack of closure he felt he'd been afforded. It was something he lived with all his adult life. Separation and a degree of estrangement from his father, Roger, meant those important conversations simply didn't take place as the years rolled on. In truth, Simon had no idea how to say goodbye, not knowing where they were laid to rest or the location their ashes were scattered. A few emails later and I was able to share the news with Simon that both funeral services and dispersions, just six-years apart in the 1970s, had taken place at Golders Green Crematorium, in North London. A full 44-years later, Simon was able to pay his respects and, perhaps, find a little extra closure.

Simon, the sick little boy and now grown man, is important. Important because it was his sickness and his mother's commitment that created renewed belief in non-related bone marrow donation. The acceptance that, in fact, any one of us can save a life if we happen to have stem cells that fit the bill.

Equally crucial were the leading medical minds of an age where aspersions and dismissals were par for the course. To trial a new approach in your job is bold at the best of times. You put yourself out-on-a-limb with the wrath of your bosses around the corner at any slip up. But a slip up, in this context, is another child's death. It wouldn't be their fault – the blood disease itself always takes ownership of this – but they would have failed to keep the child alive. Quite a tough day at the office in anyone's book.

But these pioneers were not fazed. Sure, they each employed differing tactics to reach the end goal –loudly and publicly falling out in the process – but their goals were always aligned and their motivations identical.

Jack Hobbs and John Barrett continued to professionally quarrel and duel as the years went on. On more than one occasion, either man would submit a research paper to a medical journal only for the other, sitting mere metres away down the hall, to public submit a very public letter in retort to appear in the next edition, questioning the outcomes, methodology and/or conclusions drawn. The feuding, witnessed by colleagues at the Westminster Children's Hospital, continued for a few years into the 1980s before John Barrett took his leave in 1993 and moved to the United States to head up stem cell transplantation at the National Heart, Lung, and Blood Institute (NHLBI).

At home, Jack Hobbs set up COGENT. With funding for his department being cut left, right and centre by the Department of Health[33], Hobbs took matters into his own hands by establishing The Cogent Fund in 1989, which stood for: '**Co**rrection of Certain

---

[33] The Westminster Children's Hospital, including the bone marrow transplantation unit, closed down in 1995 to be absorbed by the Chelsea and Westminster Hospital. Jack received assurances that 'his' unit would survive the move but he was never convinced this actually happened.

Genetic Diseases by **T**ransplantation'. And no, I'm not sure how he settled on this acronym either. The Professor of Chemical Immunology wished for this to bring together key findings and progress made in all types of transplantation so lessons could quickly be learned and copied.

In their 1989 symposium, they state that the "true credit" for the initiation of the first volunteer unrelated donor panel belongs to Liz Bostic and, following her death, full credit should be afforded to Shirley Nolan for growing the registry to a "world famous size". It's not possible to do justice by naming all the researchers and medical experts that advanced the field of bone marrow transplantation – this book would be double the size – but special mention should be afforded to James Watson, and his partner, nurse Jennifer Meyers. While much of the original thought around pioneering procedures at the Westminster Children's Hospital came from the mind of Jack Hobbs, Watson was able to provide the link between true academia and clinical action. It made The Gomer Berry ward at the Westminster a true centre of excellence.[lxii]

Equally important was Joe Humble, one of the founders of the Westminster bone marrow transplantation unit who, sadly, succumbed to leukaemia himself just a few years after retiring in 1980. From the moment he graduated, he started working in pathology and haematology at the Westminster Hospital and taught countless students over the years with incredible dedication and conscientiousness. He was another to marry a nurse at the hospital, Elsie May, known fondly as Ann, in 1942 and over the years was a resolute and steadfast champion of the ground-breaking work taking place inside the walls on Udall Street, in the shadow of the Palace of Westminster. Humble spotted and diagnosed his own leukaemia after taking a blood sample while test running a new piece of apparatus in the lab.

Dr Ann Barrett continued to introduce world-first radiation therapy for cancer patients. Moving to Glasgow's Beaston Oncology Centre, she teamed up with Professor Tom Wealdon where, together, they developed a mathematical formula for what they believed to be the optimal radiation dosage and delivery methodology that is still in use today. Subsequently, Dr Barrett was showered with awards, honorary fellowships and accolades in recognition of her services to the advancement of medicine, including an Order of the British Empire (OBE) in 2010. Her former colleague, Professor Ray Powles, ran the blood cancer unit at the Royal Marsden Hospital until 2003, at which point he also received Royal recognition, awarded a Commander of the British Empire CBE[lxiii]. Using detailed and hilarious stories from 60s and 70s, Professor Powles talks fondly of this pioneering time. When he started using the new immunosuppressant drug, cyclosporine, his colleagues in the U.S. were frustrated they couldn't trial any due to the strict drug approval processes. They sent for Powles; a first-class air ticket and two bags of the drug in his jean's pockets, he managed to carry the white powder all the way to the Fred Hutchinson before heading straight back to London.

Of the 4,000+ transplants he's carried out in a long career, he remembers that the first 1,000 all ended in abject failure. Before leaving the Marsden, he organised a party attended by 200 transplant donors and recipients. It was an emotional and symbolic crescendo to a prolific professional journey. With over 1,200 scientific papers to his name and lectures around the world, he is currently Chairman of the European Blood and Marrow Transplant (EBMT) Nuclear Accident Committee.

At varying times over recent years, alongside detailed reading of dry scientific papers and dusty, disjointed archive documents filed at the back of libraries, I have met with many incredible individuals to put together a greater understanding of this story. Sitting in a Tim Horton's on the outskirts of Toronto with Jim Till, no one would have known this 90-something year old is responsible for proving the functionality of a stem cell. In another coffee shop, this time in London's King's Cross station, customers wouldn't know the two people I was sitting with were doctors Mira Leigh and Caroline Lucas, crucial components to the medical team that treated of Simon Bostic, Anthony Nolan and many others back at the Westminster. Or as I waited at the entrance of Union Station, in Washington, DC, rushed and frantic commuters would not recognise John Barrett, responsible for major advancements in haematology and stem cell transplantation across the world.

Despite their differences, in style and approach, by collaborating and battling together they were able to push forward advancements in a field that had previously only experienced failure. No less worthy of praise were the parents. Here we mention a few key individuals, but interviews suggest there were many more, lesser known, that rallied for radical change and understood the bigger picture.

We are all here because of those that came before us. Our lineage is long and complicated and that's what makes each of us so complex. We've slowly understood more about those complexities and, as science and technology continue to advance, so too will our ability to tackle challenging disease. While writing this book, new scientific papers have claimed huge successes. From Professor Mel Greaves stating that a cocktail of microbes can ward off cancer in children[lxiv]; a woman deemed to be cured of HIV while her leukaemia was treated with a stem cell transplant (a full circle story, given a machine sorting stem cells originally discovered HIV) [lxv] and cord blood transplants[lxvi] becoming the new norm, easing pressure on the traditional and complicated bone marrow extraction techniques of Joe Humble, Jack Hobbs and Don Thomas.

While these advances are impactful, they do not replace the need for volunteers to donate their stem cells. Bone marrow transplantation is an effective treatment for almost every blood-based disease[lxvii] and lives still depend on strangers signing up. For all these incredible scientists, stem cell transplantation has been their life's work. At the core, blood's vast complexity has baffled and challenged for generations. They haven't done it for acclaim or celebrity – science isn't really like that – but the debt of gratitude we owe them is vast. Their radical work means should we, or others, be in the unenviable position of needing treatment for killer blood disease, we all have a substantially better likelihood of survival.

It remains a delicate balance that we still do not fully understand. As we celebrate the advancements made, and the people responsible, it's crucial to pay respect to those that have died from blood cancer. According to Blood Cancer UK charity, one in every 16 men and one in every 22 women will develop blood cancer at some point in their lives, the majority being variations of lymphoma or leukaemia[lxviii]. Today, 43 people will die in the UK due to blood cancer[lxix]. That number is around 158-people per day in the U.S. (that's one person every 9-minutes)[lxx].

A worrying downward trend transpired, in the wake of the COVID-19 pandemic saw the number of sign-ups to global bone marrow registers fall by as much as 60% compared to 2019[lxxi]. As we've seen, the greater number of people on the database the better the chance of finding a life-saving match. Even more so if you're heritage is not white-European. According to charity DKMS, a global register of stem cell donors, only 2% of the UK population are currently registered as potential blood stem cell donors, and just 13% of those on the register come from minority ethnic backgrounds (that's approximately 175,000 people, roughly 0.26% of the whole UK population).

A number of organisations are trying to coordinate public access to registers globally. DKMS and Anthony Nolan are two UK-based organisations doing this; in the U.S., BeTheMatch have a substantial database; while based out of Quebec, Mai Dueong has established a border-busting project named Swab the World, providing people in any country contact details and requirements to sign-up locally to be a stem cell donor.[34]

It's been a long road to this point. Weird and wonderful discoveries through history laying the foundations for medical advancement right up to modern day. We can now see, under the microscope, if your blood matches with someone in desperate need of it. How amazing is that.

For all those that have gone before us, all those we were unable to save, surely it's worth finding out if your unique liquid formula can save a life.

---

[34] Mai's own diagnosis came in early-2013 and, as a Canadian woman of Vietnamese-parents, Mai was told the chances of finding a suitable match were extremely unlikely and, not accepting that as an option, set about transforming this reality for people like her following her successful transplant a few years later.

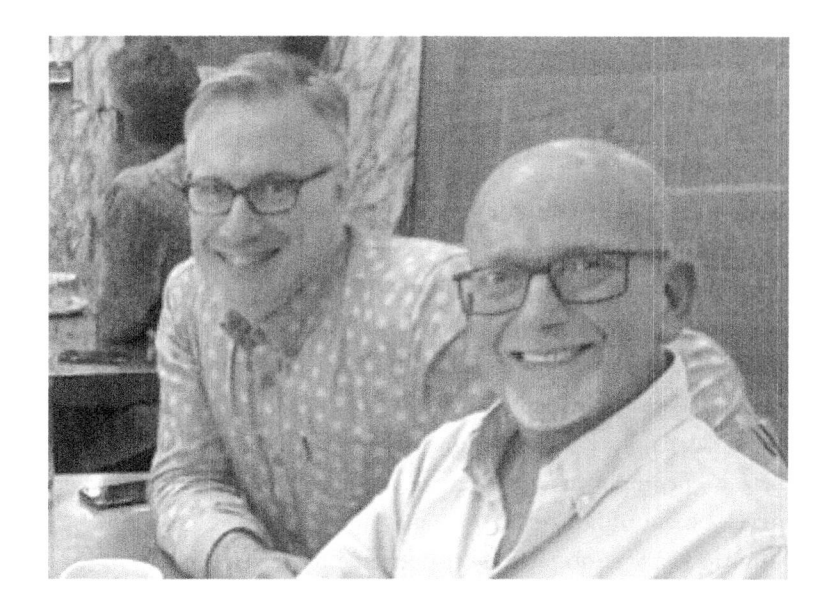

Afterword
BY SIMON BOSTIC

One of the headlines appearing in the press following my mother's death said, "look what you started, Liz!" Reviewing and working with Mike on the remarkable story of my Mother (and me) has been hard graft in itself - a challenging cathartic process. Mike has achieved something which most medical or scientific accounts do not and that is to show how scientific developments impact on human lives and how the gains achieved in science come at a huge human cost: pain and suffering caused by trials, errors, failures and successes. He has given Elisabeth Bostic, my mother, her rightful place in the pantheon of heroes who worked tirelessly for progress in research, equipment, treatments and ultimately of course, cures. I saw for myself the effect of my transplant in history when I spoke to 300 BMT survivors at a conference in Florida.

To my embarrassment, they gave me a standing ovation just for surviving. That ovation, though, was for all the survivors and their families but especially for all of those who did not make it, such as the "little angel", my older brother Andrew who I miss every day almost as much as I do my mother. And today thanks to my mother's determination to save me there are many tens of thousands of survivors of stem cell transplants.

Mike has kindly asked me to have the last word – to round off his broad, encompassing and remarkable account of the history and development of bone marrow transplants.

I must say a little about what happened afterwards.

As you have read, in spite of the incredible efforts of Profs Humble and Hobbs at the Westminster Children's hospital in 1973, I am still affected by my genetic condition, Chronic Granulomatous Disorder (a primary immune condition). Thanks to my mother's grit and steadfast determination, fighting for my chance at life and using the power of the world's media to her advantage (sometimes against the wishes of the powerful hospital management), I got that chance at survival. Having had more than 20 chest infections before I was 18 months old, the engrafted transplant did give me six infection-free years. It also gave us all a break from the terrors of life on the edge. Yes, not grafting enough bone marrow meant my BMT ultimately did not last but this experience taught the world the importance of displacing the entire host immune system. It also was the catalyst for Shirley Nolan to come to the UK in December 1973 seeking similar miracles for her son Anthony. Shirley took the baton from my mother, using the first-ever database of donors which my mother's campaigning had created, and ran with it, creating the Anthony

Nolan Bone Marrow Appeal (now the charity "Anthony Nolan"), the first register of potential stem cell donors in the world.

And yet, incredibly, I am still alive - no ordinary achievement for someone with my particular immune disorder. At 52 years, I am one of the oldest male survivors with x-linked CGD. Just as was always the case with Elisabeth, my mum – the life force is with me in spades, packaged up with a self-determined, stubborn character which just doesn't allow me to give up. The day my mum died was far and away the worst day in my life and I continue to survive the shock and tragedy of her death with each passing day. Losing that sort of a force from my life on earth has had far reaching, insidious and long-lasting effects and has been a bigger demon than any of my physical afflictions. It was not only my brother Andrew but also my mother who died as a result of this unpredictable and harsh, cruel disease.

Since birth, my future has been precariously balanced on the estimations of expert medical professionals: he won't live past infancy, then childhood; evidently, I was lucky to reach my 19th birthday and should have had another BMT. As an adult, they gave up predicting my demise and instead of putting numbers on it, resorted to vague phrases such as "your time is limited", "manage your expectations" and "do what you want to do in life sooner rather than later." One of my trusted consultants called me Lazarus due to my repeated ability to bounce back from the brink. As recently as February this year (2023) my partner of 26 years was sat down in a sideroom of an Accident and Emergency ward and told I wouldn't last the night. Mortality is staring me in the face. It has stared me down, eyeball to eyeball. I could sense its breath on my cheek. It looked deep into my soul and said, "so, how much do you love living? Is it time?"

Outliving predictions has become one of my better habits, it seems.

I have done what I wanted to do and, thanks to my adventurous and cast-iron will have lived a full and fearless life for the best part of 20 adult years. In spite of the repeated assaults on my body of all manner of infections and inflammation, time still has yet more to offer me, and the gift of life continues for the time being. I am so grateful for every moment of it – trying my best to draw the marrow out of every ounce of life still available to me. Yet whilst my hunger is great, I am not greedy – I have lived well and have been so lucky. This book has helped me to understand more clearly the huge cast of people who played crucial roles in saving my life, even long before I was born, gifting me this time. I am so grateful to them.

I hope my mum would be proud to see her efforts recognised.

I know how proud I am of her.

Author acknowledgements

Interviewees and contributors to this project, include:

Simon Bostic, Dr John Barrett, Dr Mary Horowitz, Dr Raul Scott Pereira, Professor Rainer Storb, Dr Mira Leigh, Dr Caroline Lucas, Professor James (Jim) Till, Professor Michael Gottleib, Professor Alejandro Madrigal, Dr Armand Keating, Dr Colin Steward, Professor Ray Powles, Dr Ann Barrett, Professor Leonore Herzenberg, Orin Lewis, Dr Danielli Oliveira, Mai Deuong, Professor Mel Graves, Dr Martin Raff, Natalie Amoatin, Christopher Barends, Daphne Barends, Jovana Drinjakovic, Mollie Short.

Thanks to: London Metropolitan University Library, The Wellcome Collection Library, UML Special Collections (John Rylands Research Institute and Library, Manchester University), Janet Sampson, Richinda Taylor, Alex Smith, Alan Overton, Alastair Humphries, Hannah Partos.

Special thanks to: Liz Bailey, for your constant loving support, Paul and Carol Niles, and to Liz Bostic and Shirley Nolan; for legacies that will continue to change lives.

Index

A
acquired immunodeficiency syndrome (AIDS) 144, 146, 148, 149, 190, 196
African-Caribbean Leukaemia Trust (ACLT)   192, 193
Agent Orange   173, 174, 175, 176, 177, 178, 179
anaesthetic   89, 102, 103, 187
atomic bomb   8, 12, 15, 20
B
Bari bombing   71
Barrett, Ann   97, 98, 99, 104, 105, 201, 206
Barrett, John   51, 56, 125, 126, 127, 200
BeTheMatch   203
Bone Marrow Transplantation   107
British Medical Association (BMA)   82, 84
C
Center for International Blood and Marrow Transplant Research (CIBMTR)   163, 165
chimerism   28
Chronic Granulomatous Disease (CGD)   29, 44, 45, 171
COVID-19 pandemic   203
Curie, Marie   9, 14, 92, 93, 150
cyclosporin   115
D
De Gale, Daniel   181, 182, 183, 186, 187, 191, 192, 193
DKMS   203
DNA   13, 17, 149
E
Eastwood, Susan   69, 70, 75
Einstein   9, 10, 11, 12, 14
F
fluorescence-activated cell sorting (FACS) machine   104, 148, 149
Fred Hutchinson Cancer Research Center   129, 130, 133, 136, 137, 138, 162, 166, 188, 196, 201
G
Gomer Berry Ward   24, 48, 110, 120, 127

Graft versus Host Disease (GvHD) 61, 62
Graft vs Host Disease (GvHD)   135
Graft vs Leukaemia Effect 136
Graves, Laura   162, 163, 165, 180, 188
Great Ormond Street Hospital   54, 55, 69, 70, 75, 191, 192
H
Hardisty, Roger   69, 70, 71, 75, 207
Herzenberg, Leonore   147, 148, 149, 206
Hickman line   164
Hickman Line   138
Hobbs, John Raymond 'Jack'   25, 26, 87, 89, 117, 171, 200
Hugh-Jones, Ken 45, 46, 50, 51, 110, 120, 127
human leukocyte antigen (HLA)   29, 61, 62, 105, 109, 123, 132, 138, 163, 165, 186, 194, 195
Humble, Joseph   88, 201
I
immunodeficiency 19, 26, 27, 28, 144, 149, 154
immunology   114, 116, 130, 134, 142, 148, 164
J
James, David   29, 61, 62, 109, 120, 123, 127, 155, 156, 165, 169, 194
L
Lacks, Henrietta 189, 190
leukaemia   59, 60, 70, 75, 104, 136, 192, 193, 207
acute lymphoblastic   60
luddites 101
lymphoma   59, 132, 141, 176, 178, 202
M
Mathé   18, 19, 20, 103, 104, 105, 118, 195
Meitner, Lise   12
Mond, Edith   55, 56, 90, 167
myeloma 59, 104
N
National Health Service (NHS)   50, 65, 67, 82, 83, 84, 85, 86, 151, 153
Noddack, Ida   14

Nolan, Shirley   154, 155, 170, 198, 199, 200, 206
nuclear fission   11, 12, 14, 15, 16
O
Operation Ranch Hand   173, 175
P
plasma   59, 66, 67, 104, 194
Powles, Ray   103, 104, 105, 118, 201, 206
R
radiation 95
REDOME (Registro Brasileiro de Doadores Voluntários de Medula Óssea)   195
Royal Marsden Hospital   97, 98, 104, 118, 201
S
stem cell 39, 88
Storb, Rainer   105, 131, 133, 134, 197, 206
T
The Matilda Effect   13
Thomas, Edward Donnall (Don)   24, 95, 130, 131, 132, 133, 134, 138, 139, 164, 166, 195, 196, 202
transplant
allogeneic   *27*
autologous   *27*
V
van Leeuwenhoek, Antoine 34
Việt Cộng   173, 174
Vinča   8, 16, 17, 38
Vincent Square, London   24, 50, 56, 57, 58, 90, 110, 124, 169, 199
W
Westminster Children's Hospital   26, 27, 29, 44, 45, 46, 47, 50, 52, 57, 58, 59, 61, 77, 79, 87, 88, 99, 107, 109, 118, 123, 124, 125, 133, 151, 153, 155, 156, 165, 167, 169, 171, 193, 199, 200, 201
X
X-linked disease   45
x-ray   94

Z
Zumwalt, Elmo "Bud"   175, 176, 178, 179, 180

HARD GRAFT
OUR FIGHT AGAINST KILLER BLOOD

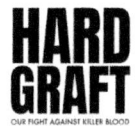

Timeline

1945 — **Elisabeth Bostic** is born.
As the atom bomb fell, mother Mollie and father Denis welcomed their baby daughter into the world in London, England

1958 — **Vinca Nuclear Accident**
An explosion at a nuclear power plant in the former-Yugoslavia means scientists desperately need bone marrow transplants from unrelated donors.

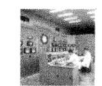

1960 — **New drugs for cancer**
With leukaemia survival rates at 0%, Dr Hardisty trials new drug mixes in an attempt to keep patients healthy for longer.

Only 1-in-10 children with blood disease live to adulthood

1963 — **Discovering the source of life**
Scientists Till and McCulloch demonstrate the utility of the 'stem cell'. A new understanding is born about how to generate fresh blood

1968 — **First successful bone marrow transplant**
Performed between siblings, Dr Robert Good is the first person to successfully graft stem cells

1970 — **Andrew Bostic** is born: first child of Elisabeth, and her husband Roger.

Younger brother, **Simon**, soon follows (born in 1971).

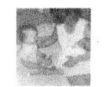

1973 — **World's first unrelated bone marrow transplant**
Simon Bostic becomes the first human to receive a successful bone marrow transplant from a stranger

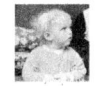

1974 — Understanding the potential of unrelated transplants, the world's first bone marrow registry launches in the UK in 1974... starting out in a basement broom cupboard

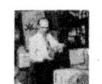

1999 — Daniel De Gale becomes the first Black British recipient of an unrelated bone marrow transplant. 9-in-10 children with blood disease live to adulthood

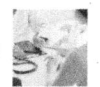

HARD GRAFT

References

_____

[i] Mitchell CD, Richards SM, Kinsey SE, Lilleyman J, Vora A, Eden TO. Benefit of dexamethasone compared with prednisolone for childhood acute lymphoblastic leukaemia: results of the UK Medical Research Council ALL97 randomized trial. Br J Haematol 2005;129:734-45.

[ii] Matloub YH, Angiolillo A, Bostrom B, Stork L, Hunger SP, Nachman J, et al. J Clin Oncology 2007;25(18S):9511

[iii] William Potter, Djuro Miljanic, Ivo Slaus, Published in The Bulletin of the Atomic Scientists, http://www.bullatomsci.org/
March/April 2000, Vol. 56, No. 2, pp. 63-70 © 2000 The Bulletin of the Atomic Scientists

[iv] Dahl, Per F; From Nuclear Transmutation to Nuclear Fission, 1932-1939; CRC Press, 1 Jul 2002

[v] https://www.world-nuclear.org/information-library/current-and-future-generation/outline-history-of-nuclear-energy.aspx

[vi] https://www.youtube.com/watch?v=6UvbdidT-qM

[vii] https://www.nobelprize.org/prizes/lists/all-nobel-prizes

[viii] https://www-danas-rs.translate.goog/vesti/drustvo/misterija-vinca-akcidenta/?_x_tr_sl=sr&_x_tr_tl=en&_x_tr_hl=en&_x_tr_pto=sc, Nenad Kovacevic, 17th May 2012

[ix] https://www.signalsblog.ca/the-story-of-the-first-bone-marrow-transplant/, Jovana Drinjakovic | Sep 15, 2016

[x] 'Rainbows through the Rain': many details in this section are from the unnamed book written by Liz Bostic's mother, Mollie Short. These were shared by Simon Bostic.

[xi] Oxford Dictionary of National Biography 2005-2008 edited by Lawrence Goldman;
https://books.google.al/books?id=nbGcAQAAQBAJ&pg=PA550&lpg=PA550&dq=the+cogent+trust+hobbs&source=bl&ots=FWA3eBuAbk&sig=ACfU3U1BIsdl1iVsP2EKq1F-JPpg4bSG0A&hl=en&sa=X&ved=2ahUKEwju657EhPzkAhUOC-

wKHWFLDRgQ6AEwAHoECAYQAQ#v=onepage&q=the%20cogent%20trust%20hobbs&f=false

[xii] Piller, G.J. (2001), Leukaemia – a brief historical review from ancient times to 1950. British Journal of Haematology, 112: 282-292. https://doi.org/10.1046/j.1365-2141.2001.02411.x

[xiii] BECKER, A., McCULLOCH, E. & TILL, J. Cytological Demonstration of the Clonal Nature of Spleen Colonies Derived from Transplanted Mouse Marrow Cells. Nature 197, 452–454 (1963). https://doi.org/10.1038/197452a0

[xiv] Thomas Adam, Transnational Philanthropy: The Mond Family's Support for Public Institutions in Western Europe from 1890 to 1938, Palgrave Macmillan Transnational History Series, Springer 2016

[xv] Thomas Adam, Transnational Philanthropy: The Mond Family's Support for Public Institutions in Western Europe from 1890 to 1938, Springer, 26 Jul 2016

[xvi] https://www.jstor.org/stable/3856342

[xvii] https://collections.nlm.nih.gov/bookviewer?PID=nlm:nlmuid-101584649X142-doc#page/1/mode/2up

[xviii] https://www.ferris.edu/HTMLS/news/jimcrow/question/2004/june.htm

[xix] Out for Blood; Anastasia Kirby Lundquist. CreateSpace Independent Publishing Platform (July 24, 2014)

[xx] https://www.nhsbt.nhs.uk/who-we-are/a-history-of-donation-transfusion-and-transplantation/

[xxi] https://www.youtube.com/watch?v=r8D7AwfJUkY&t=60s

[xxii] Dante Alighieri (1265–1321). The Divine Comedy

[xxiii] The US signed the protocol in 1925 but the Senate didn't ratify this until 1975.

[xxiv] How a WWII Disaster—and Cover-up—Led to a Cancer Treatment Breakthrough - HISTORY

[xxv] Dobbs, Michael (1998-11-30). "Ford and GM Scrutinized for Alleged Nazi Collaboration". *The Washington Post*. Retrieved 2009-06-01

[xxvi] GOSH01349_Breakthrough_guide_Cancer_complete_lores.pdf

[xxvii] Hardisty, Roger M. et al. "Vincristine and Prednisone for the Induction of Remissions in Acute Childhood Leukaemia." British Medical Journal 2 (1969): 662 - 665.

Published 14 June 1969

[xxviii]

https://media.gosh.org/documents/Legacy_Cancer_Breakthrough_Guide_booklet.pdf

[xxix] https://www.independent.co.uk/news/obituaries/obituary-professor-roger-hardisty-1240925.html Tuesday 23 September 1997

[xxx]

http://news.bbc.co.uk/1/hi/events/nhs_at_50/special_report/119803.stm, Wednesday, July 1, 1998

[xxxi] Opinion of close colleague, Colin Steward, revealed during interview, 10th Sept 2021

[xxxii] Somewhat less well known is the fact that forty years earlier, someone else had made the same accidental discovery. Abel Niepce de Saint Victor, a photographer, was experimenting with various chemicals, including uranium compounds. Like Becquerel would later do, he exposed them to sunlight and placed them, along with pieces of photographic paper, in a dark drawer. Niepce thought he had found some new sort of invisible radiation and reported his findings to the French Academy of Science. No one investigated the effect any further until decades later when Becquerel repeated essentially the same experiment on that grey day in March 1896 - This Month in Physics History (aps.org)

[xxxiii] https://resource.rockarch.org/story/philanthropys-fight-against-tuberculosis-in-world-war-i-france/

[xxxiv] https://associationofanaesthetists-publications.onlinelibrary.wiley.com/doi/pdf/10.1111/j.1365-2044.1980.tb03951.x

[xxxv] Provincial Medical and Surgical Journal 1847;s1-11:330

[xxxvi] Davy, Humphrey; Researches, chemical and philosophical; chiefly concerning nitrous oxide or dephlogisted nitrous air.

[xxxvii] GB 133 MMM/12/2, Manchester University Archives, Special Collection

[xxxviii] Early opposition to anaesthesia, https://associationofanaesthetists-publications.onlinelibrary.wiley.com/doi/pdf/10.1111/j.1365-2044.1980.tb03951.x

[xxxix] Title: Medical Essays, Author: Oliver Wendell Holmes, Sr., Release Date: August 16, 2006

https://www.gutenberg.org/files/2700/2700-h/2700-h.htm

[xl] British Society for Immunology: 1976 Spring Meeting, London (Wed 21, Thurs 22, Fri 23 April)

[xli]

https://www.fordlibrarymuseum.gov/library/document/0036/pdd750904.pdf

[xlii] C. D. Buckner, R. B. Epstein, R. H. Rudolph, R. A. Clift, R. Storb, and E. D. Thomas, "Allogeneic Marrow Engraftment Following Whole Body Irradiation in a Patient with Leukaemia," *Blood* 35 (1970): 741-50

[xliii] R. O. Hickman, C. D. Buckner, R. A. Clift, J. E. Sanders, and E. D. Thomas, "A Modified Right Atrial Catheter for Access to the Venous System in Marrow Transplant Recipients," Surgery, Gynecology and Obstetrics 148 (1979): 871-75

[xliv] https://www.ncbi.nlm.nih.gov/pmc/articles/PMC1470620/

[xlv] 'And the band played on', Randy Shilts

[xlvi] On average a white blood cell has a diameter of 12 - 17 μm (micrometre). A human hair is around 50 μm.

[xlvii] Fluorescence-activated Cell Sorting (FACS) | Sino Biological

[xlviii] Derry JM, Ochs HD, Francke U (August 1994). "Isolation of a novel gene mutated in Wiskott-Aldrich syndrome". Cell. 78 (4): 635–44. DOI:https://doi.org/10.1016/0092-8674(94)90528-2

[xlix] https://rarediseases.info.nih.gov/diseases/7895/wiskott-aldrich-syndrome

[l] Interview with Shirley Nolan, Credit: ITN, Editorial #812980822: https://www.gettyimages.ae/detail/video/bone-marrow-transplantation-at-westminster-hospital-news-footage/812980822

[li] https://www.theguardian.com/society/2002/jul/17/voluntarysector.guardianobituaries

[lii] Woman's Magazine, 1983: Kathy Watts

[liii] Magnuson, Ed; A Cover-Up on Agent Orange?; Time Magazine, Sunday, June 24, 2001

[liv] Quote from Zumwalt's Z-gram: "I sincerely believed that I was philosophically prepared to understand the problems of our Black navy men and their families, and until we discussed them at length, I did not realize the extent and deep significance of many of these matters".

[lv] Ex-Admiral Zumwalt Claims Manipulation On Agent Orange, Bill McAllister, Washington Post, June 27, 1990

[lvi] Washington HA, editor. *Medical Apartheid: The dark history of medical experimentation on Black Americans from colonial times to the present.* New York: Random House, Inc; 2006.

[lvii] Skloot, R: The Immortal Life of Henrietta Lacks

[lviii] Batts, Denise Watson (May 10, 2010). "Cancer cells killed Henrietta Lacks - then made her immortal". *The Virginian-Pilot.* pp. 1, 12–14. Archived from the original on May 13, 2010. Retrieved February 20, 2021.

[lix] 'Saving Children's Lives', Westminster Children's Hospital promotional brochure, at London Metropolitan Library, year unknown.

[lx] Fee E, Brown TM. Michael S. Gottlieb and the Identification of AIDS. Am J Public Health. 2006 Jun;96(6):982–3. doi: 10.2105/AJPH.2006.088435. PMCID: PMC1470620.

[lxi] https://www.theguardian.com/society/2002/jul/17/voluntarysector.guardianobituaries

[lxii] https://history.rcplondon.ac.uk/inspiring-physicians/james-graham-watson

[lxiii] https://cancercentrelondon.co.uk/consultant/prof-ray-powles-cbe/

[lxiv] The Observer, Robin McKie, Sun 30 Dec 2018 04.00 EST: https://www.theguardian.com/science/2018/dec/30/children-leukaemia-mel-greaves-microbes-protection-against-disease

[lxv] https://news.sky.com/story/first-woman-to-be-cured-of-hiv-with-stem-cell-blood-cancer-treatment-say-us-scientists-12543370

[lxvi] Cord blood is found in an umbilical cord, connecting a baby in the womb to the placenta, both being a rich source of stem cells. If a mother agrees to donate her baby's cord blood, the procedure is safe and simple.

[lxvii] Appelbaum, Frederick MD, Living Medicine; Don Thomas, Marrow Transplantation, and the Cell Therapy Revolution Mayo Clinic Press (29 Jun. 2023)

[lxviii] https://bloodcancer.org.uk/news/blood-cancer-facts/

[lxix] https://bloodcancer.org.uk/news/blood-cancer-facts/

[lxx] https://www.lls.org/facts-and-statistics/facts-and-statistics-overview

[lxxi] https://news.sky.com/story/steep-decline-in-potential-stem-cell-donors-may-make-life-threatening-blood-cancers-harder-to-treat-charities-warn-12781626

Printed in Great Britain
by Amazon